UNDERSTANDING

M.E.

THE PHENOMENON OF MYALGIC ENCEPHALOMYELITIS AND ACUTE ONSET POST VIRAL FATIGUE SYNDROME

Dr David G. Smith

Robinson Publishing
London

Robinson Publishing
11 Shepherd House
Shepherd Street
London W1Y 7LD

First published 1989
Revised and updated 1991

British Library Cataloguing in Publication Data
Smith, David G.
  Understanding ME
  1. Man. Myalgic encephalomyelitis
  I. Title
  616.8'3

ISBN 1 85487 105 6

Typeset by Selectmove Ltd.
Printed by The Guernsey Press

Acknowledgements

I should like to take this opportunity to thank all the M.E. sufferers whom I have had the privilege of meeting over the years, and from whom I have learnt a great deal. Thanks are also due to my wife Isama, for her patient understanding during the writing of this book, and to Lynn Batty for her dedicated typing abilities and for her forbearance towards me despite the number of times we have had to rewrite it. I have, however, thoroughly enjoyed doing it, and I have found that trying to communicate the many fascinating features of this disorder has helped me to crystallize my thoughts about the facts of which we can be certain and to keep an open mind about those which as yet remain a mystery.

CONTENTS

PREFACE to the PAPERBACK EDITION

Understanding M.E. was first published in May of 1989. Then, I indicated that the field of M.E. was 'a vast and rapidly expanding one' and that 'my opinions will change as I am prepared to keep an open mind to any new medical evidence on any aspect of this disease'. There is no doubt that I have changed my mind in a number of cases. There have been some exciting new developments in understanding the mechanisms of how enterovirus infections become persistent, and of how the symptoms of this disease are probably generated from an area at the base of the brain called the hypothalamus. But the most surprising change is my understanding of the origin of the fatigue and realization that there is probably very little wrong with the skeletal muscle. I hope that I will continue to keep a broad-based approach and an open mind, as when that becomes closed it will be time to stop, though one's mind must never be so open as to allow one's brain to fall out. I hope that you find this revised edition of greater help and understanding.

Introduction

M yalgic encephalomyelitis (M.E.) is a term referring to a series of unexplained fatigue syndromes. Being such, it is not a diagnosis, but a label for a collection of particular symptoms giving rise to an illness of yet undetermined proportions and causes, and there are probably many different disease processes giving rise to these symptoms.

There is, however, at least one disease process lasting for many months, or even years, which has been reported throughout the world for several centuries. It has occurred in sporadic epidemics in different geographical locations and in small or large groups, and consists of a syndrome of chronic muscle fatigue, vague malaise and ill-health, and of other varying recurrent symptomatology, especially referring to the central nervous system, with symptoms and problems suggestive of a psychiatric disease. These outbreaks have been extensively documented and explained, and can be found no better described than in Dr Melvin Ramsay's book *The Saga of the Royal Free Disease*.

The association of these outbreaks with a viral cause, and specifically with the enterovirus Coxsackie B, has been intimated for many years. Scientists in America are inclined to the Epstein Barr virus as the offending viral organism – the virus which is usually assocated with the clinical phenomenon of glandular fever, or infectious mononucleosis.

Researchers in Great Britain, Australia and New Zealand have suggested many alternative causes – notably candida albicans, but also food and chemical intolerance, allergy, mineral and vitamin deficiency, environmental factors, and mercury poisoning. There are still further, more obscure, theories.

These disease complexes and their various forms currently travel under the name myalgic encephalomyelitis (M.E.) but because of a global lack of understanding of the disease processes involved, several different collective names are used, such as benign myalgic encephalomyelitis, epidemic neurasthenia, sero-negative glandular fever, chronic Epstein Barr virus syndrome, Bornholm's disease and Royal Free Disease. Where epidemics occur in different parts of the world, they acquire the name of the geographical location for instance Iceland disease, Tapanapi flu, Akureyri disease and Los Angeles Flu, and, because of increased media attention, the illness has gained more populist names such as 'yuppie flu'. It would seem likely, because of the similarity of symptomatology, that these various styles of 'viral' disease share a common process. However, the name used will continue to vary until a specific clinical definition is applied, or the causative factors are clearly identified.

Within this book I have laid down two specific disease process definitions which will narrow the origination of myalgic encephalomyelitis down to particular viral causes and allow the introduction of the clinical phenomenon of acute onset post viral syndrome. This will, I believe, present disease processes with which the medical profession can identify and will form the basis for future research, until, or unless, some other clinical definition can be sought in the light of new scientific facts.

In Britain much research, victim support and dissemination of information is generated by the M.E. Association, a registered charity which has proved itself more than capable of providing this umbrella support. In this country, therefore, it would seem to be advantageous to retain the name of myalgic encephalomyelitis to focus medical attention and to prevent the confusion caused by variation in the nomenclature.

Seldom within medicine have the attitudes to one disease process been so argued over and the causative agents so hotly disputed. The greater proportion of informed medical opinion still believes that the illness is primarily psychiatrically based, and denies any organic substrate. As for the rest, it lies between maintaining an open mind to the problem, and the minority, like myself, who believe that the disease process is purely organically and virologically based, especially when dealing with the specific clinical phenomenon of acute onset post viral fatigue syndrome (AOPVFS).

Within the group of disease processes that M.E. displays I have developed a specific interest in AOPVFS and this book is written with the specific aim of furthering understanding of that. It also, however, covers several aspects of M.E. – its symptomatology, the clinical course, diagnostic investigations, current research virology, immunology, other research programmes and the management and treatment of its manifestations.

The book also discusses possible future research areas, and the support programmes, aims and objects of the M.E. Association; it contains the majority of official medical advice given by that association, but also includes very personal views. I hope that the information will be upgraded and republished frequently, as the field of M.E. is a vast and rapidly expanding one.

The medical advice given, apart from my own, is taken from many sources. My opinions will change, as I am prepared to keep an open mind to any new medical evidence on any aspect of this disease. That being said, the advice contained herein is the best currently available and I hope you will find the book helpful and informative.

1
THE HISTORY OF THE M.E. ASSOCIATION

The M.E. Association is a relatively young charity which sprang from one woman's illness and her endeavours to find out what was wrong, not only with herself, but with others who shared similar symptoms.

In 1973, Pamela Searles, the M.E. Association's present Secretary, developed an illness which appeared to have been the result of some kind of virus infection. When her condition did not improve she went to see several doctors within her home area of Essex but they were unable to tell her what was wrong. After spending several months searching for an answer, she was eventually referred to a consultant microbiologist at Basildon Hospital – Dr Betty Dowsett, now retired. After discussing Pamela's symptoms and doing several investigations, Dr Dowsett suggested to her that she was suffering from what was known at the time as Royal Free Disease.

Dr Dowsett told Pamela to listen to the radio the following day, when Dr Celia Wookey would be broadcasting a programme on Royal Free Disease; together with Dr Wookey and several other doctors, Dr Dowsett was forming a medical study group to look into the causes of this illness.

During that broadcast, Dr Wookey said that she would be prepared to send questionnaires out to people who thought they had a similar disorder, and by looking at these questionnaires she would try her best to help solve some of their problems. The returned questionnaires were in fact studied by Dr Wookey, Dr Dowsett, and Dr Melvin Ramsay, a recently retired consultant from the Infectious Diseases Unit at the Royal Free Hospital who had been consultant in charge of that unit at the time of the 1955 outbreak which gave the disease its name.

At one particular meeting with Dr Dowsett, Pam Searles met a retired nursing sister called Joan Pearce, who wanted to do some form of medical voluntary work. Dr Dowsett suggested that Pam and Joan might like to start a local group for sufferers of Royal Free Disease and so the Royal Free Disease Association was born.

In the following months, Joan and Pam visited people in the Essex area who had replied to the questionnaires to discuss the various problems and symptoms, and the ways in which they could all help one another. A local committee was formed and the participants' involvement grew to the extent that they began to handle letters and questionnaires from all over the country.

Some 250 questionnaires had been received after Dr Wookey's broadcast, and because of this large number Pam Searles thought it would be a good idea to call a meeting in central London. At the end of 1976 a meeting was held at Friends House, a large building just opposite Euston Station, and the problems of the disease were discussed by the many people who turned up.

The Association ran as a self-help organization for nearly two years, guided for the most part by a group of interested medical practitioners, known as the Medical Study Group – some of whom felt that they also had the disease or certainly something like it. They formed the main background for the medical direction which the Royal Free Disease Association would take in the future.

At this stage, Dr Peter Behan, a consultant neurologist from the Glasgow Institute for Neurological Sciences, approached the Association for some financial funding for a particular research programme. Dr Behan had already been doing research on M.E. for a number of years and, finding specific research funds difficult to obtain, asked the Association for £5000.

It became apparent that the self-help Association would find itself in some legal difficulties in raising money and donating it to medical research, so the treasurer at that time, Mike Debenham, suggested that the Royal Free Disease Association should become a registered charity. This it duly did in late 1979, the trustees all being husbands of Royal Free Disease sufferers.

The Medical Study Group, and in particular Dr Ramsay, were not keen on the name Royal Free Disease, preferring myalgic encephalomyelitis; consequently, the charity was set up under the name of M.E. Association. The charity's first task was to raise the £5000 for Dr Behan which, after a large amount of effort at local level, it succeeded in doing.

Medical interest in M.E. was developing quite rapidly in the early 1980s and the Medical Study Group, chaired by Dr Ramsay, guided the medical approach for a number of years. Dr Ramsay was invited by the M.E. Association to be their president, a post which, at the age of 87, he still holds.

For the first two or three years of the M.E. Association's existence, things remained relatively quiet. The membership increased slowly and the majority of the members had not received a medical diagnosis. However, they all had symptoms which were similar and problems which mirrored those printed in the initial M.E. Association Newsletters and pamphlets. They were therefore a self-diagnosed group. By 1983/4, the membership was approximately 500, fund-raising was a constant struggle, and a vast amount of work was done by relatively few people. The input of effort was enormous.

The fund-raising for research programmes continued, but apart from Dr Behan's work there was in fact little interest in research. As there was hardly any new information about the illness, publicity in the press and on radio and television was hard to come by.

The vast majority of medical opinion still believed that M.E. was a non-diagnosis, or that it did not exist, and if it did, it was psychiatrically based. Advice from the M.E. Association on the clinical management of the disease, especially that of physical rest, was not accepted, and indeed was sometimes ridiculed.

In 1986 M.E. suddenly hit the headlines. Mention of it was made in 'Agony Aunt' columns of women's magazines and the quality Sunday papers ran whole page editorials and articles on people suffering from M.E. The disease began to 'take off'. This was partly due to the work of Professor James Mowbray of St Mary's Hospital, Paddington, who, in 1979, had begun research into M.E. His important virological contributions began to bear fruit in 1986 and 1987, when the disease became more respectable and accepted.

Doctors began to make the diagnosis, were more amenable to accepting an organic origin, and would refer patients to the M.E. Association rather than leaving them to discover it for themselves.

People with similar symptomatology who had been undiagnosed, misdiagnosed or simply mishandled continued to seek an answer for their strange fatigue syndrome and the membership doubled each year from 1984, with ever-larger sums of money being raised for research. The Association's need for official premises led to the acquisition of a shop with a large flat above it in Stanford-Le-Hope, Essex. Donated goods are sold in the shop, very much along the lines of the Oxfam principle, while upstairs the flat has been converted into offices of one large and two smaller rooms. It is already too small, as the Association has two full-time secretaries and nine part-time salaried staff, including an accountant, and a move to larger premises seems inevitable.

At the time of writing the membership is 12,000, increasing at the rate of 150 per week. I believe that there are over 100,000 people in Great Britain with this disorder, and clearly this is going to present a logistical problem to the M.E. Association. However, it is a challenge that they are looking forward to, as the majority of this very large number of people still do not know what is wrong with them, and probably 90 per cent are still being told that their disease is within their mind. We will have the job of getting through to them and their medical practitioners as M.E. becomes more widely heard of and understood.

The function of the M.E. Association

The work of the M.E. Association is divided into three main areas. The first is to locate possible sufferers and to offer them support through a network of local groups; and to provide assistance in obtaining a diagnosis and access to medical testing not widely available elsewhere. The second is to promote research into treatment and cure, and the third is to spread information about the illness so that the general public, the medical profession and the caring agencies become aware of its effects.

In addition, the Association gives advice to sufferers on how to cope with their own personal difficulties. Letters received from its members, and reports from volunteers within the Association, have helped to identify many needs, among them the feelings of isolation and frustration experienced by patients which are compounded by difficulties in achieving a diagnosis and anxiety and depression due to the effects of the illness. Financial problems are another worry for sufferers – eligibility for benefit has appeared not to depend on the severity of disability so much as the knowledge of the examining doctor and his acceptance or otherwise of M.E. as a physical illness. This difficulty also extends to the availability or otherwise of services such as home helps etc.

The real strengths of the Association's support to sufferers lies in the local self-help groups, which are established all around the country. It is within these groups that members can share experiences with those who are facing the same symptoms and the same difficulties. Many groups organize meetings with speakers who talk on all aspects of M.E., both medical and social, and some hold fund-raising events to support the central organization and, most importantly, research.

There is also a volunteer telephone counselling service which is manned by sufferers who are experienced in counselling. It is a confidential service operating five evenings a week with some day time cover, and is extremely popular with members. Further important support is provided by the welfare section, which offers individual help in negotiations with the DHSS, employers, education authorities, social services and other organizations with whom members may encounter difficulties.

The Association has circulated a booklet called *Diagnostic and Clinical Guidelines for Doctors*, the joint work of several doctors who have the longest service and perhaps the best knowledge in the field of M.E. A medical pack is available to any doctor who applies for it, with the aim of reducing the misdiagnosis and/or mishandling which is frequently the lot of the M.E. sufferer.

My own involvement with the M.E. Association

Ten years ago, I was Medical Assistant at a large psychiatric hospital, doing eight sessions a week, as well as running a small, single-handed general practice in a village in Essex. My patients numbered about 1,000, one of whom was Pamela Searles, who asked if I would look after her on a private basis. She told me that she had M.E. and presented me with a booklet on the subject; like the majority of doctors at the time, I had never heard of it. She also gave me the M.E. Association's bibliography, and I read all of its references. Her illness had originated from a virus infection which she had had some several years prior to my meeting her, and she was still badly affected by typical M.E. symptomatology.

Some of the treatment I offered her was relatively successful and she felt a great deal better; I suppose it was because of this, and because I had lent a sympathetic ear, that several other women with M.E. came to see me as well. If they had disease processes other than M.E. I had variable success in treating them, but as to the underlying problem and the syndrome that they suffered from, I, like others, drew a blank.

By the end of the year, I had accrued twenty or so of the M.E. Association's sufferers, which at the time totalled some 300. The Association asked me to become their Medical Advisor, and so I started to learn more about M.E. by reading all available material and by meeting medical exponents of the disorder. They usually referred to a viral start, and to post viral syndrome, especially in association with the Coxsackie B viruses.

The amount of work that this project was beginning to generate was prodigious, and I had to make a choice as to whether I would continue working within the local hospitals and general practice, and the National Health System as a whole, or whether I should resign and commit myself wholly to looking at the clinical picture of M.E. and trying to start research work in general. I had become quite absorbed in M.E. and it really was not much of a decision to make, as I found it such an exciting and stimulating problem and I felt I had to be in the 'front line'.

I developed a working contract with the M.E. Association, and they funded me with a retaining salary, initially for one day a week. My terms of reference were to act as their Medical Advisor, to write articles for the M.E. Newsletter, to correspond with doctors, and to further the understanding of M.E. by lectures, discussions etc. The rest of my time was taken up in work on patients with the syndrome. There was unfortunately no way that I could be funded under the

National Health, and in the absence of any research monies, this had therefore to be on a private basis.

I thus became peripatetic, able to see anybody anywhere, to try to sell my ideas and various pathological samples to interested parties, and to try to pick their brains – and, where appropriate, twist their arms – to help me find out more about this mysterious disease.

So far, I have had no trouble along these lines – it seems that interested parties do not require very much in the way of arm twisting or ear bending in order to become involved, and it is these people that I must thank for our current knowledge.

My first expert advice was that obtained from Dr Douglas Bainbridge, Consultant Immunologist at the London Hospital, Whitechapel. I went to see him initially because of his known expertise in looking at white cell function and his laboratory's skills in analysing auto-antibodies.

In the early stages, I spent a lot of time talking about the disease with Dr Betty Dowsett, Consultant Microbiologist at Basildon Hospital, and was then introduced to Dr Eleanor Bell, who runs a reference laboratory for enterovirus studies. They suggested I should meet Dr Bob Gamble at Epsom Public Health Laboratory, who was an expert in Coxsackie virus infections, and Professor Banat Valar at St Thomas' Hospital, London, who had developed a new antibody assay for Coxsackie B viruses.

However, I think that most of my thanks must go to my mentor Professor James Mowbray, who stimulated all of my initial enthusiasm and drive and without whom I would not be in my present position. I met him in the early stages when, as Medical Advisor to the M.E. Association, I went to a meeting in Cambridge, where post viral syndrome was the subject under discussion. I was seated at the back of the hall, one row in front of Professor Mowbray, who was next to Professor Banat Valar. Dr Behan was giving the talk, but I constantly heard over my shoulder the words 'circulating immune complexes – viral antigen – persistent enterovirus infection – IgM'. Not understanding what these terminologies meant, I approached Professor Mowbray during a lunch-break at the meeting and asked whether he would assist me by applying some of his newly developed specific tests on my patients. He was kind enough to agree and, as most M.E. sufferers are aware, his laboratory is now responsible for the provision of the first national blood testing facility available through the M.E. Association.

By this stage I had seen a great number of patients with M.E. but, because of the diversity of symptomatology and clinical presentation, and the lack of an identifiable start, I really did not know what I was looking at, except to suggest that they all had a rather non-specific fatigue syndrome. However, I suddenly became aware of an emerging clinical picture. There was a group of patients who seemed to tell exactly the same story, to have exactly the same type of symptoms and, for the first time, they appeared to have a specific clinical phenomenon. I saw several patients who had undoubtedly been fit and well, with no history of any other significant disease process or illness in the past, until they had developed an apparent respiratory tract infection – a 'flu-like illness', from which they said they had never fully recovered. Some had a lot of the other M.E. symptoms, others very few; some were desperately unwell, and the disease had destroyed the quality of their life. Others were only slightly ill, but all of this group complained of one common symptom – that if they indulged in what was, for them, a lesser than usual amount of physical activity, they suffered an undue degree of general muscular fatigue from which it took an unreasonable time to recover. It was from this particular group of patients that my interest in post viral syndrome developed, and it was this that was to form the basis of the clinical work to come.

To me, then, at that time, the clinical picture was quite clear. I felt that there was a definite physical disease with an unknown cause, and although I could not tell my patients what was wrong, or what was going to happen to them, they clearly had a disease process, initiated by some kind of virus infection, that was continuing to make them unwell.

This had a beneficial effect on these patients because at last someone had a possible explanation for their illness. Somebody understood their problems and did not simply dismiss their symptoms as psychiatric, which appeared to be the general rule, prior to them seeing me. It was also beneficial in that some of them had been convinced that there was something else physically wrong, and that doctors who had told them there was nothing wrong were clearly missing something – something possibly more serious. They could not accept or believe that they were basically psychiatrically ill. I was surprised to find that some 50 per cent of them thought they had a serious, as yet, undiagnosed disease, such as multiple sclerosis or a brain tumour. Therefore my telling them that they had post viral syndrome, and that they would probably get better, seemed to help enormously

Many members of the medical profession who did not agree that M.E. was organically based would strongly criticize what I had done. If the patient had been told that his or her disease process was primarily psychiatric, as had frequently happened, then the psychiatrist would say that my approach was totally counterproductive, as it would simply compound the patient's reluctance to accept the psychiatric diagnosis that he or she had been given; and that if he or she continued to believe in an organic origin, supported by me, he or she would never, or only infrequently, get better.

Such medical practitioners would also say that patients of this type continued to do the rounds until they eventually found a doctor who would tell them what they wanted to hear. I have also had it suggested to me that the diagnosis of M.E. is made by a medical practitioner who has an altered approach to the disease – i.e. the doctor who diagnoses M.E. is as sick as the patient! A consultant neurologist from Kent was quoted as saying that he considered a particular case of M.E. as 'near-delusional self-deception' and that M.E. was 'a figment of the imagination both on the part of the patients who think they are suffering from it and the doctors who make the diagnosis'.

Psychiatrists suggested that we should discontinue further research into M.E. and other forms of post viral syndrome since the investigation itself might 'increase the severity of the symptoms and the signs'. Their view was that medicine should return to the pure psychiatric approach, which I found spectacularly blinkered and non-progressive.

Along similar lines, I saw one consultant neurologist's letter to a general practitioner which said of his patient, 'I have told her that she has M.E. – while condemning her to a life of chronic ill health, it will at least get her off the medical merry-go-round!'

I have heard some tragic stories of medical mishandling and wrongful diagnosis which placed excessive pressure upon the patient and the family, with resulting loss of employment, break-up of marriages, and generally unnecessary despair. It is worth recounting some case histories to illustrate the harm that can be caused by ignorance of, and scepticism about, this illness.

In June 1987 I received a letter from a consultant physician who knew of the work that I had been doing, and indeed we had corresponded on points of mutual concern. Now he had a case in which he wanted me to take an interest.

Debbie was fifteen and a half, and the physician felt that there was little doubt about a clinical diagnosis of post viral syndrome. She had been too ill to go to school for about eighteen months, and the letter contained the information that increasingly acrimonious exchanges had taken place between the education department, her doctors and her parents, and she was now threatened with a care order. The referring physician was clearly sympathetic to her plight and asked if I would see her with a view to doing muscle biopsy studies, to confirm the diagnosis.

In August 1987 Debbie came to see me, accompanied by her parents, and her story went like this:

Debbie was described as being a perfectly fit and happy only child, having never been significantly ill until the first week of February 1986, when she went to school in normal health. At 3.00 p.m. she suddenly felt rather hot, ill, headachey, tired, and nauseated; on her return home she felt more unwell, and was quite ill for about a week. She was off her food, she had a very sore throat, a high temperature, but symptomatic improvement was noticed, and a doctor was not consulted.

While not fully recovered she felt well enough to return to school, but when she reached there, she felt hot, dizzy, very unsteady, and started to sweat. She felt more unwell as the day progressed and by the end of the afternoon felt totally shattered. This continued for a week until, in the middle of one afternoon, she felt and looked so ill she was told to go home. She walked home a mile and a half in the freezing cold, arriving in a very poor state with stomach pains, diarrhoea and extreme fatigue.

This time a doctor was called, and he felt that she had gastro-enteritis, for which there was no specific treatment, although he prescribed an antibiotic for her continuing sore throat. After a further three days she again improved and, though still not quite right, returned once again to school.

A further week went by, with the continuing symptoms of feeling hot and cold and sweaty, with a sore throat and abdominal discomfort. The diarrhoea stopped, but she started to develop pains in her legs and arms, and her muscles began to ache. She had since failed to make a full recovery.

At the time of this interview she was still clearly unwell, being pale and drawn. Her parents did most of the talking, explaining that she had had a rough time, and she was very wary of doctors. After some while she was able to tell me that she still felt ill, just as she had when she still had the flu eighteen months previously. Her major symptom appeared to be a profound tiredness and lethargy, she felt sick most of the time, and she suffered headaches which would always come when she did anything physical and which were unrelieved by aspirins and paracetamol.

She felt hot and cold, although each time her parents took her temperature it seemed to be below normal. She described pains in virtually every muscle of her body, which were made worse by walking. She could not talk too much either, because it gave her a headache and made her feel ill. She did not like company, because she could not follow the conversation of more than one person at a time; two or three people confused her, and she became emotional and frequently cried. She found some of the school work that she had been given to do at home very difficult, because she could not read a sentence and follow its meaning; she would read the same line over and over again, but it would not sink in. She could not concentrate, finding even simple television programmes difficult, and she did not much like the television or radio because the noise upset her.

She would go to bed early and get up late, sleeping much more than usual, but even when she was up during the day she still felt exhausted and sleep did not seem to satisfy her desire to rest. On occasions she felt rather claustrophobic at home, and would go out for a walk; after only a few hundred yards the colour would drain from her face and she would suddenly feel nauseated and more unwell. It was clear from the description of the severity of her various symptoms that Debbie was not well enough to go to school.

My immediate reaction was that she had a classical case of acute onset post viral fatigue syndrome. With this in mind I enquired about Debbie's previous health, both physical and mental, and there did not appear to have been any problems. She was not taking medications of any kind and there was nothing in her parents' lives that might suggest either a physical or psychological problem. There seemed to be a good family relationship.

Her father then described the difficulties the family were having with the local county council, which was making moves towards taking Debbie into care.

In June 1986, about five months after Debbie's original infection, she was admitted to a local hospital, where it was thought that she had a urinary tract infection and some kind of virus problem, the symptoms of which were made worse by her periods. She was then referred to a child psychiatrist, who decided that there was nothing sinister in her medical symptomatology, and that the answer probably lay in disharmony between Debbie and the school.

Debbie and her family had several appointments with the psychiatrist and these did not go very well, as Debbie's mother kept insisting there was something physically wrong. By December 1986 the psychiatrist was suggesting a period of assessment and observation in an adolescent unit, and he felt that Debbie could cope with full-time schooling.

At this stage Debbie's mother took a whole series of articles and pamphlets on M.E. to the referring physician. While he agreed that this was a possibility, he also pointed out the controversy about whether M.E. was physically based or just a psychological problem; for his own part, he did not come down on either side of that fence, but sat on top and kept an open mind. From a medical point of view that would have been fine, but the psychological aspect was still vigorously pursued.

The psychiatrist then wrote to the physician, saying that if in January 1987 there was no clear medical reason why Debbie should not return to school, further steps would have to be considered.

The education department then became more involved, and there was a case conference on Debbie which was attended by the psychiatrist, education officers, welfare officers etc. At this meeting, Debbie's mother put forward the possibility of M.E. and this was discussed; however one member of the case conference stated that the 'parents are determined on finding an illness and persuading Debbie that she has it'. The psychiatrist suggested that Debbie's mother seemed to want Debbie to be dependent on her.

At the end of this meeting, it was declared that 'if the parents refuse to cooperate, care proceedings should be sought, which may encourage the parents to be more positive'.

At the end of February Debbie was taken to an alternative therapist, a registered homeopath, who diagnosed post viral syndrome and wrote a letter to the Education Authority to this effect. One month later, by the end of March 1987, it was suggested that Debbie might be 'encouraged to go to a physically handicapped school'. In June, a place was found at this school for the physically handicapped and the county education officer wrote at the end of June that 'the local education authority is mindful of its statutory obligation to provide Debbie with education, and will view, with grave concern, any continued absence of schooling. The local education authority will therefore give serious considerations to any necessary measures to ensure her continued education. I am sure that as concerned parents you will support this'.

Debbie's mother, still convinced that there was something physically amiss, sought legal advice and contacted their GP again to ask for another opinion. The GP referred them to the consultant of my acquaintance, who immediately diagnosed post viral syndrome and effected a referral to myself.

Over the next few weeks I sent letters to all the medical personnel who had seen Debbie, and asked for their opinions and for photocopies of any relevant findings. Meanwhile, I instigated the serology and the various tests that I had available, and I was able to demonstrate an intermittently persistent enterovirus and also the presence of immune complexes. While this did not prove M.E. it did demonstrate a physical abnormality that would support the clinical diagnosis of an organic type of post viral syndrome.

I then composed a letter to the education authority, saying that Debbie was still physically ill, and that this court order should cease. I sent a copy of the letter to the initial physician involved, and to the psychiatrist, asking for their comments first; the physician replied that it was a reasonable interpretation, and he accepted my judgement that it was possibly a physical disorder. I did not get a reply from the psychiatrist.

In October 1987, I wrote to the education department pointing out that the consultant who referred Debbie to me, her GP and of course myself all diagnosed post viral syndrome and believed it to be a physical illness, and I asked that the court order should be removed. This was in fact what happened and no further pressure was put upon Debbie, who, by the end of October 1987, was sixteen years old, and could have left school anyway!

This particular story is quite a common one in children. When the consultants who assess the situation do not believe the possibility that post viral syndrome or M.E. is a physical disorder, they either sit on the fence or, even worse, make a purely psychiatric diagnosis, so that the children become something of a football. They do not have control over the consequences of their own illness because they are under age, and the education authority feel the children are not being educated because of some fictitious or self-induced disease that is probably a combination of abnormal illness behaviour on the part of the child and some kind of emotional disorder within the mother and or the father.

This problem shows the importance of establishing how much of post viral syndrome is physical and how much is psychological, and it also demonstrates the need for physicians, psychiatrists and welfare agencies to keep an open mind so that a multi-disciplinary approach can be adopted. It is horrible to end up in such a mess as in this case, with the parents seeking legal advice to fight the powers that be. Debbie fully recovered by January 1990, and she has remained well since and is training to be a Nursery Nurse.

I first met Mark in the early part of November 1987, when he was twenty. This was an unusual case in that I saw him very early on, and although I would not normally make a diagnosis of post viral syndrome in under six months, there was no doubt that he was extremely ill.

He described himself as being a fit, healthy and active young man, until some two months previously. One particular Sunday evening, after he had been very short-tempered all day, he went to bed early feeling tired and woke up in the small hours feeling so unwell that he literally could not get out of bed. He had a piercing pain behind both eyes; he ached all over as if he had been hit from head to toe; he had a raging sore throat, a very high temperature and felt exhausted.

After a couple of days of improving symptomatology he felt a great deal better and went out shopping, but at the end of the afternoon his symptoms returned in a matter of moments. Again he felt dreadful, his muscles ached all over, he felt that he could not stand up, his sore throat came back. He went straight back to bed, where he spent the next few days. The sore throat disappeared but everything else stayed exactly the same; he continued to feel awful, with widespread muscle aches and pains, and a constant headache. He could not concentrate and he became very nervous; indeed, he admitted to being quite convinced that this degree of illness was going to lead to death.

He went to see his doctor, who told him that he had got flu; blood tests a week later were negative, and glandular fever tests were normal. He went to an ear, nose and throat specialist, who did not find anything wrong. His symptoms began to worsen and he did not feel that he had the strength to get out of bed; every time he stood up he felt dizzy. He was sleeping twenty-three hours a day, and this situation persisted for about six weeks.

At this point Mark's uncle got to hear of his illness and, knowing my particular interest, asked that I see him. This I did, and from a clinical point of view I felt that this was an acute onset post viral fatigue syndrome.

I examined Mark, and there was nothing of note to find, except that his hands and feet were very cold. I told him that I felt this was post viral syndrome and that at the moment he should continue to rest until there was some slight improvement, at which time some graduated exercise could be introduced.

I instigated a whole series of investigations, and they were totally unhelpful. His Epstein Barr virus serology showed that he had never been exposed to an EBV infection. His enterovirus studies were normal, as were his routine biochemistry and virology, so there was no evidence of any specific active virus.

By this time eight weeks had passed and his employers were clearly a little concerned, but fortunately very supportive. I explained the situation to the company doctor and was optimistic in my prognosis. I felt that I was rather sticking my neck out here, because as yet Mark had not improved. However, by the time he came back for his results, he was a good deal better. He looked less unwell and less haggard, he had a bit more energy and had actually gone down to the snooker hall and had a game with his pals for about an hour. I was encouraged, and told Mark to go for a pleasant stroll each day and come back in a week.

On his return the following week he was brighter still, so I told him to attempt a little more each day unless it caused a setback. When he managed this without suffering any ill-effects I suggested he exercise a little bit more than he should, to push himself. This was again successful, so I felt that in the absence of knock-on fatigue the next day there was every likelihood that his post viral syndrome had abated. Consequently, I encouraged him to do more and more, and within a further five months he was totally well.

Susan first came to see me in September 1987, by which time she had been ill for three years, with no improvement. She was working at the time the illness struck, and had always been a fit and healthy young woman with no significant problems of any type. She was living happily with her parents and was planning to marry her fiancé of several years' standing, with whom she had bought a house six months earlier.

She remembered it being a nice summer, with long warm evenings, but unusually for her she had been coming home tired from work for no obvious reason. Instead of going out in the evenings she had been going to bed at about 9.00 p.m.

One particular evening she went to the pub with her fiancé and had a glass of wine, which tasted very peculiar. She went to bed early with a strange sensation in her throat and woke the next morning feverish, with hot and cold sweats, extremely swollen and tender glands in her neck, and a feeling of being extremely tired. The symptoms progressed, and she felt generally ill for the next week, with a continuing sore throat, aches and pains, and a generalized malaise and tiredness.

Susan went to see her doctor, who told her that she had a virus infection, and she had blood tests, including a Paul Bunnell test for glandular fever which gave a positive result. She continued to suffer from malaise, tiredness and lethargy and a further Paul Bunnell test again proved positive. She was told that she had a persistent type of glandular fever, and that it was not unusual for this particular infection to go on for some time.

Her symptoms not only persisted, they deteriorated. She constantly went to see her doctor complaining of being exhausted, with recurrent sore throat, stiff and aching muscles, and peculiar muscle cramps – she would go very stiff, and her muscles would be very sore on movement. She continued to feel feverish, although her temperature was always normal. She had a headache most of the time, her hands and feet were cold, she was getting nightmares, and she did not sleep very well. She felt extremely agitated and worried, although about what she was not sure. After a month she became depressed, irritable and very moody, especially premenstrually. She felt persistently overtired despite long periods of sleep, her memory began to deteriorate, and her concentration fell off remarkably.

A month or so into her illness Susan had started to lose her appetite, finding food was unpleasant, and she developed a stomach upset with intermittent diarrhoea. She noticed that chemicals and food made her feel nauseated. Her eyesight started to blur, light upset her eyes, and very soon she found that she was hardly able to do anything. Every time she went for a walk, probably less than fifty yards, the muscles in her arms and legs started to ache and twitch, and her legs turned to jelly.

Because of the remarkable consistency of her symptoms and the fact that they did not seem to improve at all, her doctor continued taking Paul Bunnell tests which, after nearly a year, became normal. Her doctor then suggested that there was nothing now wrong with her, and that she should try to push herself and go back to work. This she did, but she managed only a few hours before she felt so ill that she had to go home; when she pushed herself the thing that she noticed most of all was that the nightmares became worse. Her rest and sleep became more disjuncted, and she felt more tired the next day and the day after.

A few more months went by like this and it was suggested that she should see a psychiatrist. He said that there was nothing psychiatrically wrong with her, certainly nothing that could cause her symptomatology, and that there was something physically wrong.

By July 1987 there had been no improvement, all of her tests had been negative now for some eighteen months, and both Susan and her doctor were at a loss to know what to do. She was referred to the Hammersmith Hospital where she saw a physician who told her that there was nothing wrong with her; she went back to see the same psychiatrist who kept telling her that she was physically ill. Finally, Susan went to a doctor in Wimpole Street who told her that she had post viral fatigue syndrome, and suggested that she should contact the M.E. Association.

Susan's degree of disablement was considerable and what worried me was the fact that she had an almost static disease that was now over four years old. She was very depressed and became very upset when I said there was probably little that I could do for her, apart from suggesting graduated exercises and a further psychiatric referral in order to see whether a tailor-made antidepressant might help with the psychological aspects of post viral syndrome.

I sent her to a colleague who specializes in this area and he suggested some medication, agreeing that all her anxious, depressive and neurotic symptoms were associated with her viral disorder. However, she seemed little, if any, improved by the antidepressants and in fact they seemed to upset her. Her virology and routine blood tests were, as expected, normal, but her specific virology for the Epstein Barr virus, the virus responsible for glandular fever, was still positive. She showed the serological evidence of reactivation and presumably the illness at the beginning was that of a true Epstein Barr virus.

This was one of the very few cases I had as yet seen where I could be as near certain as possible that this disease was due to the Epstein Barr virus and thus it seemed to me that glandular fever could go on to produce a post viral fatigue syndrome. This was to revolutionize my thinking over the next months.

At the time of writing Susan is still ill, and there has been no significant improvement. We must find a cure for this disease, since at present there is little hope we can offer to people in her position, and I am convinced that we will have one, or at least a very efficient treatment programme, within the next five years even if our research continues only at the current low level of technology and expenditure. We also need to find first very hard scientific evidence of an organic basis to, and a well-defined clinical picture of, this disease to overcome the scepticism and even downright antagonism which is found among many of the medical profession.

To find this evidence, one has simultaneously to develop two approaches. The first one is to define the clinical disease and the second to develop tests to show that what is going wrong in that group of patients is specific only to that group. This requires a stance which is quite unusual in medicine, and that is to start with the clinical problem and develop the appropriate technology around it.

A test for a disease must, in the perfect situation, be easily reproduceable, reliable and accurate, and must produce a clear-cut positive result, in the whole of that defined clinical picture. The test should have been negative before that disease process started, and should become negative again if the clinical disease process abates or is successfully cured. It should never give a positive result in a normal healthy person, and should not be positive in any other disease process.

Tests like this are very seldom available, and there is usually some overlap and interpretation required. However, some of the tests and investigations which we in the medical profession who have taken an interest in M.E. have developed are finally leading towards the desired specificity.

2
WHAT IS M.E.?

The name myalgic encephalomyelitis literally means: *mya* – muscles; *algic* – painful; *encephalo* – brain; *myel* – nerve; *itis* – inflammation. A disease, then, suggesting painful muscles, and inflammation of the whole of the nervous system. The more we learn about this condition the less appropriate the name would seem to be, because not all people with M.E. have painful muscles, and certainly none of them have any evidence to date of any brain, nerve or central nervous system inflammation.

Major symptoms which are found in M.E., such as loss of memory and concentration, are not incorporated in the name, nor is the variety of symptoms suggested. However, I do not feel that it is time to propose yet another change of name, although I do suggest that the disease definition of M.E. is tightened up.

As the name implies, however, the disease is certainly a collection of symptoms that affect all of the central nervous system and muscles and do not have a predilection to go for one specific area, or side, more than another. Because of this collection of symptoms, M.E. must clearly contain a number of different disease processes as possible causes. It is, then, a syndrome, rather than a specific diagnosis.

In this respect it is rather like 'flu', which is also a syndrome, and which both the general public and the medical profession would similarly understand to consist of vague aches and pains, sweats, malaise, raised temperature, feeling hot and cold etc. The diagnosis of 'flu' would not tell you the cause, which is often assumed to be a virus, and there are many viruses which will give rise to that collective symptomatology of flu. These include the true influenza viruses, but rhinoviruses, adenoviruses, enteroviruses and others are all capable of causing an upper respiratory tract 'cold' and a 'flu'-like illness. However, the syndrome of 'flu' is far more specific than the syndrome of M.E.

M.E. is characterized by a set of primary major symptoms, the most important of which is the pathognomonic symptom of excessive muscle fatigue, which has an extended period of recovery. Other main symptoms include myalgia (muscle pain), loss of concentration and memory problems. There also tends to be a general feeling of tiredness and malaise, and a non-specific feeling of being profoundly ill. Major symptoms that are not invariably present also include a recurrent sore throat, glandular tenderness, anxiety, depression, emotional lability and a loss of facial colour, often associated with cold hands and feet.

Then comes a collection of secondary minor symptoms which are very variably found from one patient to another. They include headaches; dizzy spells; visual focusing problems; disturbed sleeping patterns and nightmares; chest pain; palpitations; a feeling of shortness of breath; gastro-intestinal upset, including indigestion, flatulence, distension and wind (collectively termed 'irritable bowel'). One certainly can go on from there with a list that is extensive. The symptoms are sometimes quite bizarre and have little reasonable medical explanation, especially as they tend to vary from time to time, all of which contributes to continued medical disbelief.

The beginning of the disease process differs. It can have a very sudden and acute onset, where a person who is normally fit and well is suddenly struck by the collection of symptoms listed above. Alternatively, the problem can come on insidiously, with no definitive start. Some patients say that they cannot remember ever having been well, and that the symptoms have been there for as long as they can remember.

If this clinical picture is mixed with a more recognized medical condition, such as bronchial pneumonia, acute appendicitis or a road traffic accident, then perhaps the less important occurrence of what appears to be a minor cold or flu-like illness is lost historically as the start of the problem, and medical practitioners are bemused by the profound collection of symptoms appearing after what would be a medically simple event from which a normal recovery should have occurred.

The clinical picture of M.E. is one of fluctuation. Patients can have good days and bad ones, good weeks, months, or even periods of relatively good health extending into years, without ever having quite recovered from their 'flu'; they may be struck down again at any time by a recurrence of symptoms. Unfortunately, others find no respite from their problems, and they continue with an unremitting chronic disease. The majority, fortunately, note that the symptoms gradually disappear or improve, and many are eventually asymptomatic when their disease process dwindles and recovery occurs. It is, I believe, only the minority who remain ill for what appears to be a lifetime.

There is very little in the way of objective clinical evidence of illness to support the patient's usually extensive symptomatology. Examination of the patient produces little clinical finding and there are certainly no focal or localizing signs. The disease is global, affecting the whole of the body without any predilection for one side or another.

Routine, but often very extensive, investigations have failed to find any abnormality to show that there is a disease process. These investigations have included, for instance, haematology, biochemistry, virology, x-rays, cardiographs, brain scans, NMR scans and ECGs and none have revealed an abnormality which could justify the severity of the disease the patients complain of.

My belief is that M.E. and some of its subgroups are entirely physically based. That being the case, how can one explain these extremely variable global symptoms in the absence of substantive medical proof?

My reasoning is very simple, and that is that medicine just has not got there yet. It is not equipped with the investigative powers and techniques to explain these phenomena. Within M.E. we are probably working with functional abnormalities of cellular metabolism, and the way in which cells work or don't work, the problems, abnormalities and lesions lie at a sub-cellular level.

Medicine has got to grips with the understanding of large tumors, which can be seen and felt and cut out. Equally, it understands gross inflammatory diseases of muscles, blood vessels, etc; it has explanations for problems at the level of bacteria and viruses. However, it is only just beginning to understand immune dysfunction, chronic virus illnesses and abnormalities, and the problems within the nucleus and gene. It is at this level that I believe the abnormalities lie, so the reason why our tests do not show anything wrong in M.E. patients is simply because we have not yet developed the correct tests.

I can understand and sympathize with the despair of the doctor who, in a busy general practice or an overcrowded out-patients clinic, is confronted with a patient seeking yet another opinion on a collection of symptoms which are seemingly endless. M.E. patients will sometimes complain only of their more marked or important symptoms, because they feel that if they make a full confession of all their problems they will instantly be labelled neurotic or even downright insane. Unfortunately, if they take their symptoms out of context they often find those problems being specifically, and inappropriately, investigated. Then, with the negative results that usually occur, there is still no answer. If, on the other hand, the patients mention all of the symptoms and the fact that they have had them for fifteen years – and that there does not appear to be a start, or a middle, and certainly no end, and that it is all getting worse – the temptation for the physician to say that they are hypchondriacal or polyneurotic must be very strong.

I have heard many physicians' answers, and they include, 'I think it is your nerves.' 'You are just depressed.' 'I cannot find anything wrong – isn't that good news?' 'I will write and tell your GP all about it.' 'What do you expect? You are over forty! It's your age!'

Without a clear, universally accepted clinical definition of M.E. that can be readily identified by all medical practitioners, the concept of M.E. will necessarily mean many things to many men. The vast majority of disease processes are clearly and very specifically defined by the World Health Organisation (WHO), so that doctors throughout the world, when seeing a patient, know exactly what they are looking at, and know also that all other doctors throughout the world have the same standard of reference. They can thus discuss the problems, investigations and treatment while being miles or even continents apart.

Without such a definition, this clearly cannot be the case in M.E. The medical profession is going to be constantly at a disadvantage, and will be discussing the disease at cross-purposes. This is compounded by the fact that without such a disease definition, one doctor who makes a diagnosis of M.E. will not be able to discuss the problem with any doctor making the same diagnosis, because they are possibly, even probably, looking at totally different things.

Physicians studying the M.E. syndrome have developed a multitude of sophisticated investigations, and there are suggestions that there are various, and variable, abnormalities to be found. However, most of the tests are currently non-specific and one cannot apply a non-specific test to a non-specific disease process and expect to get anything other than total confusion.

Such confusion is particularly well demonstrated in the extremes of alternative medicine, where practitioners apply non-scientifically established 'tests' and then pronounce a diagnosis of M.E. This will inevitably lead to further alienation of the M.E. sufferer and the M.E. Association from mainstream medicine. I, as the Association's Medical Advisor, have tried to maintain a hardline approach to developing and recognizing acceptable disease concepts and criteria and to the development of scientific tests. I must therefore necessarily divorce myself, and guide the M.E. Association away from, the further extremes of alternative diagnostic capability and remedies.

I have seen a lot of people with so-called M.E. and listened to a lot of symptoms and stories, and I still do not know what M.E. is. To clarify the situation, I believe that it is correct to adopt the perception of M.E. as recently recognized by the Department of Health and Social Security.

In the latter part of 1987 written questions were made by MPs to Edwina Currie, then the Junior Minister of Health. Her reply made it clear that the DHSS and her Majesty's Government accepted M.E. as a disease process, and that in itself was a tremendous step forward.

3
ACUTE ONSET POST VIRAL SYNDROME

The majority of my early M.E. patients were self-diagnosed, and there was no doubt that there was an enormous collection of pathology which was initially confusing.

Certainly the symptoms were similar, not infrequently identical, but it slowly emerged that there was a subgroup of people who were fit and well until they were suddenly struck by an illness which was very suggestive of a virus infection, from which they had not recovered.

The indication that it was initially a virus infection was that they had frequently developed an acute sore throat, with a temperature, malaise, and widespread aches and pains. Sometimes they had clearly caught it from another member of the family, or there was a lot of it going around at the time. In the absence of any other reasonable explanation, this would constitute a starting point for defining post viral syndrome.

By the time I had seen twenty or so such cases, I was impressed that despite the often quite large amount of psychiatric symptomatology the underlying illness appeared to be a physical one. The patients had problems with their muscles, which were painful, and they expressed the feeling that they were often not able to think properly, they could not concentrate and their memory was poor. It did not appear to me to be a psychiatric type of illness; I believed them to be suffering from the lingering effects of a 'virus illness'.

Before defining what I took as being the clinical picture of post viral syndrome, I should like to propound my view as to why the medical profession should look at post viral syndrome as an organic disease process.

At the time that I was studying these patients, in the early 1980s, the medical profession, to a greater extent, believed that post viral syndrome was primarily a psychiatric problem. It had been part of their medical training that after a virus infection patients were left with a depressive illness.

I cannot accept the argument some doctors put forward that post viral syndrome just does not exist. It clearly does exist; patients are sitting there saying that they feel ill. Since it is a recognizable illness, the argument must be in what form it exists. Is it physically based, is it a psychological problem or is it possibly a mixture?

I maintain that all acute onset post viral syndrome is primarily physically based. Although it contains a lot of variable psychological symptomatology, it is not primarily a psychiatric disease. I have therefore adopted a totally different standpoint from the traditionally accepted medical view.

I believe that the main reason for the primary psychiatric diagnostic stand maintained by the medical profession is that it has an overall view of total knowledge on any one subject – in other words, if the examination reveals no obvious physical problem or localizing sign, and the tests applied are negative, the patient is probably not physically ill and therefore must be psychiatrically ill. Instead of saying, 'I do not know what is wrong', doctors will say that it is nerves, anxiety or depression, because medicine does not like to have no answers to the problem.

Medicine has a very polarized attitude between physical disease and psychiatric illness. There is very little grey in the middle. Not only that, but in the case of post viral syndrome there a great number of substantial symptoms which would strongly suggest a psychiatric disorder, for example, anxiety, depression, sleep disturbance, loss of appetite and the irritable bowel type symptoms. If the physician's physical examination and tests are negative, it is not unreasonable for him to say that the illness is primarily psychiatric. Or is it?

Why not adopt the other approach as I have done, and say that this virus has caused a physical disease with a lot of psychological symptoms; that the muscle and joint aches and pains, cold hands, feet, etc. are in fact physically based and not psychologically so; and that the psychological symptoms are a feature of the disorder, rather than a cause. After all, there are many organic diseases in which the psychiatric symptoms dominate the clinical picture. Nobody would suggest that the ageing of the brain, as seen in pre-senile dementia, is psychological, but its psychiatric symptomatology is often horrendous. Other diseases of primary central nervous system dysfunction that have psychological problems include: the inflammatory diseases of the brain, such as meningitis and encephalitis; hardening of the arteries, causing arteria sclerotic senile dementia; the confusion seen in cardiac failure and respiratory disease; oxygen deficiencies of anaemia; vitamin deficiencies; toxic side-effects of drugs; and malignant deposits in the brain. They give rise to organic brain syndrome symptoms, neurotic symptomatology of anxiety and depression, confusion and altered consciousness. Many are reversible; when the disease is cured the symptoms go away, and this is also the case in post viral syndrome. Where spontaneous recovery does occur, all the symptoms of post viral syndrome disappear, and the patient returns to a normal healthy life.

It can be seen, therefore, that post viral syndrome certainly does not set a precedent. Medicine does accept that psychiatric symptoms occur in primary physical disease, but it is still clear that because the symptoms are global, intangible and subjective, and because they still defy investigative procedures, the physician continues to lean towards the psychiatric diagnosis.

Establishing the study group

Over a period of time I accrued a group of approximately one hundred people, the majority of whom were female, who were fit until they had gone down with an upper respiratory tract infection from which they had not recovered. All complained of a specific symptom of excessive muscle fatigue, which they experienced after being exposed to what to them appeared to be a trivial amount of physical activity, and which took an undue length of time to recover from. I sometimes found relatively minor, but interesting, sighs, such as a slightly raised pulse, cold hands and feet, and muscles tender to the touch. In some I gained the impression that their musculature was slightly weakened, but on the whole, they could, at any one moment in time, exert a full normal force. They had a lot of other symptoms as well, but none of them, on full physical examination, could be found to have any localizing signs or problems that could answer their general symptomatology. For instance, they did not have high blood pressure, heart problems, or central nervous system signs. Other routine tests excluded thyroid problems, rheumatoid arthritis, or other biochemical or haematological abnormalities that could possibly explain their symptoms. If any such diseases were found, they were excluded from further study.

If the patients had had an appendicectomy done several years before, or had their tonsils and adenoids out, or suffered from minor aliments that could not be considered to be contributing to their current problems they remained in the study group; but if they were suffering from other chronic diseases and were taking medication, say for high blood pressure, they would not be further studied. The people who were well before a virus infection and who did not have anything else significantly wrong with them formed the basis of our definition of post viral syndrome and constituted a group which would be further 'pruned' for our study of the disease.

The definition of acute onset post viral fatigue syndrome

In June 1987 Professor James Mowbray and I gave an address at a postgraduate meeting in Manchester on M.E. and the evidence for persistent enterovirus infection in that syndrome. We had received a particularly frosty reception – the audience were unanimous in their view that the whole disease process was hysterical! They did not believe a word of what we were saying and I felt that this was partly attributable to my poor contribution at the talk in that I was not able to give a hard clinical definition of what we were looking at.

It became apparent that it was going to be of paramount importance that we should define a very specific disease process that could be recognized by doctors and universally accepted as a platform from which we could later work and expand. This is the definition that we developed: *That disease process lasting for six months or more, occurring in an initially essentially fit and healthy person, who historically suffers from a flu-like illness associated with malaise and pyrexia, suggestive of a viral aetiology; who continues to suffer from undue muscular fatigueability which has an extended period of recovery; and in whom is often associated myalgia, loss of concentration and short-term memory, the symptoms for which have no other reasonable explanation; and in whom, on physical examination, no hard localizing signs can be demonstrated.*

This disease definition excluded a lot of people who have chronic infective processes caused by viruses which are of the slow and insidious onset type, and other types of post viral syndrome. However, if we could start somewhere, using a hard kernel specifically defined and investigated, and accepted by the medical profession, we could then develop tests around that clinical phenomenon, so that those tests could be retrospectively applied to the less well-defined disease processes and demonstrate specific abnormalities within that group.

It was this particular disease definition that formed the basis of the study to come.

4
THE STUDY

By the end of 1985 I had seen approximately 150 people who believed that they had M.E. Because of the lack of understanding of M.E. there would clearly be many different disease processes occurring within this group.

I did not wish to develop any kind of preconceived ideas as to what symptoms I would find in M.E. or AOPVFS except that of the typical muscular fatigue and its extended period of recovery. I simply assessed each patient individually and made a diagnosis as best I could from their story and from the clinical picture. They fell quite clearly into three categories.

First, typical AOPVFS sufferers. This group consisted of people who gave a story of being absolutely fit and well until one day, possibly even one hour, when they had started to develop an acute upper respiratory tract type infection, a viral type of illness, with symptoms which included a sore throat, feeling hot and cold, sweating, a raised temperature, a non-specific malaise, and widespread muscle aches and pains. Some could remember catching it from a friend or relative. In some, this virus infection had developed into a localized symptomatology requiring further investigation.

For instance, a few had developed a very severe headache at the beginning and there had been a question as to whether they were suffering from some kind of viral meningitis or encephalitis. They had spent a few days in hospital having appropriate tests and had been told that they had had some kind of central nervous system virus. Others developed chest pains, and some a typical viral pericarditis as demonstrated by ECG and other tests. Others had had labyrinthitis (inflammation of the middle ear), bronchitis or viral gastro-enteritis.

These specific symptoms and the initial disease had usually settled but the patients were left with the variable symptomatology from which they had never recovered.

The second category constituted a group who were in most respects very similar to the first group. Their current symptoms were identical in that they had the same type of malaise, muscle fatigue, aches and pains, body fatigue etc., but there did not appear to be the clear-cut story of a virus so typical of Group 1. They too had been fit and well until a particular period in time, but the onset was over weeks or months, usually starting with an increasing malaise, tiredness and non-specific ill-health.

It seemed that they had exactly the same disease process as the first group, but presenting features and story were totally different. Within this group, however, no other reasonable explanation was forthcoming, other than that they were possibly suffering from the same phenomenon as Group 1 but with a different start. These were defined as slow onset M.E. sufferers.

The third group presented a story which would be very much more difficult to interpret, even impossible to unravel clinically. The symptoms did not fit M.E. or, on clinical examination, there were clearly other possibilities. These included overt psychiatric disease, multiple sclerosis, rheumatoid arthritis and hypothyroidism. One man had a past history of a known pheocromacytoma (a tumour of the adrenal gland), another subsequently had a pituitary tumour, and there were two cases of Danazol poisoning (a drug used in the treatment of endometriosis).

This last group was as large as Groups 1 and 2 put together. I decided Group 3 should act as a control for symptomatology in the questionaire only when looking at the interpretation of specific blood tests that were going to be applied to the first two groups.

Apart from these three categories I thought it would be reasonable to look at another group of people who were to all intents and purposes normal, and who would describe themselves as being fit and well – a group numbering twelve in all, which included myself, members of my staff and their relatives.

Finally, a fifth group was included. During the study programme, a colleague of mine had found an outbreak of a true para-influenza virus amongst his patients and I used sixteen of them to look at the virology and immunological abnormalities that might occur in this group, who would then be seen as suffering from an acute flu-like illness. All of them made an expected normal recovery within a period of about a month at the longest.

I then drew up a questionnaire which, without being too extensive, would give me information on most aspects of the disease, its clinical presentation, possible aetiological factors, clinical course and symptoms. I incorporated some questions with regard to possible food intolerance, chemical intolerance or candida albicans, features that I had discussed with Dr Jonathan Brostoff, a consultant immunologist and allergist.

The format was such that it could be put on to a computer database, most of the questions being yes/no or 0–3, 3 being very severe and 0 being absent. It thus gave some degree of quantitative response.

Before the study and questionnaire could be started it was necessary to establish the clinical status of each of the groups and to do baseline haematology and biochemical investigations. If any significant physical or biochemical abnormality was found in either Group 1 or Group 2 that could in any way contribute to their symptomatology, they were necessarily excluded from further study. Only relatively minor abnormalities were allowed, such as skin cysts, varicose veins, piles, ingrowing toenails etc. The criteria applying to Groups 1 and 2 did not apply to Group 3, in which any clinical abnormality would be allowed.

In all those studied, basic haematology and biochemical screening included the following: a full blood count, white cell count, and differential; T and B cell subsets; an ESR and a RAHA. Biochemistry included a 10 channel SMAC, a CPK and a TSH. Autoantibody screening included an ANA, skeletal muscle antibodies and central nervous system antibodies. The specific tests that were applied for virological assessment are more fully explained elsewhere, but included a general viral screen, a Coxsackie B IgM antibody assay by Elisa and IgM circulating immune complexes.

All of the above routine screening, excluding the specific virology and immunology, had to be normal in the members of Groups 1 and 2 for them to be included in the study. Three patients, when looked at in this fashion, produced minor abnormalities requiring their withdrawal. The blood tests of a routine nature that I did had probably been performed at least once elsewhere and, almost without exception, those investigated elsewhere had actually been through the medical wringer. Many had had far more extensive investigations done, including cardiography, chest x-ray, bone scans, muscle biopsies, EMGs, brain scans, CAT scans and EEGs, and all of these had been noted to be normal.

Where these particular tests had been performed, or where the patient had previously been hospitalized or referred to me by a medical practitioner, I wrote for relevant information, so that not only did I have results on the testing that I had instigated, but a great deal of further information as well. If there had been any significant abnormal finding in any of these specialist investigations, the patient was also deemed not to be eligible for the purposes of this study.

The only exception was those patients who had been told that their illness was psychiatrically based. However, where the patient had seen a psychiatrist, I again wrote for relevant medical information. Only if the patient had had significant psychological problems prior to the onset of their illness were they considered for exclusion from further study.

By now we had carefully selected patients in Groups 1 and 2 with suitably matched control groups. The problem was, what to do now? So far all I had done was to confirm that one could not find anything wrong with the patients, either clinically or using the very specialized investigations currently available.

Clearly, I was in a catch 22 situation, in that I had to know a little bit about what was wrong with the patient in order to define which tests should be applied. But was the technology to find out what was wrong with these people available, or did it have to be developed?

The answer to that question really is a little bit of both. Historically and anecdotally AOPVFS and M.E. have been associated with the enteroviruses and thus it was clear that I should look at the availability of new scientific facilities for testing patients to assess their virological responses and immunological status. Other studies had also suggested that there were abnormalities in the skeletal muscle. Patients complain of muscle fatigueability, muscle aches and pains and brain dysfunction, so I would have to approach various muscle experts to apply their specific investigative powers and technology.

I was quite certain that some of the investigations that I would look at would be negative, but this would at least narrow the field of enquiry.

Personal questionnaire on acute onset post viral fatigue syndrome and myalgic encephalomyelitis

Date:

Surname:

Christian names:

Date of Birth: **Sex: Male/Female**

Address: ....
....
...............................**Postcode:**..........

Occupation: Current   ....
Past 1   ....
Past 2   ....

Work

Employed full time	Y/N
Employed full time but off sick	Y/N
Unemployed	Y/N
Unemployed as result of this illness	Y/N
Redundant	Y/N
Retired	Y/N
Retired early	Y/N

Retired early as result of this illness	Y/N
Medically retired	Y/N
Medically retired as a result of this illness	Y/N
Considering retirement	Y/N
Part-time	Y/N
Part-time as result of this illness	Y/N
Part-time as result of other medical reasons	Y/N
Housewife	Y/N
Housewife needing extra help social or domestic	Y/N
Housewife needing extra help as result of this illness	Y/N
At school	Y/N
Off school as result of this illness	Y/N

Marital status

Married	Y/N
Single	Y/N
Single as result of this illness	Y/N
Separated	Y/N
Separated as result of this illness	Y/N
Divorced	Y/N
Divorced as result of this illness	Y/N
Widowed	Y/N

Family history:

Spouse with this illness	Y/N
Parents with this illness	
Siblings with this illness	
Children with this illness	

Leave above blank
or with a number.

Family history of:	Relation 1	Relation 2	Relation 3
1 Asthma	Y/N	Y/N	Y/N
2 Eczema	Y/N	Y/N	Y/N
3 Hayfever	Y/N	Y/N	Y/N
4 Rhinitis	Y/N	Y/N	Y/N
5 Migraine	Y/N	Y/N	Y/N
6 Thyroid disease	Y/N	Y/N	Y/N

7	Irritable bowel	Y/N	Y/N	Y/N
8	Pernicious anaemia	Y/N	Y/N	Y/N
9	Drug sensitivity	Y/N	Y/N	Y/N
10	Aspirin sensitivity	Y/N	Y/N	Y/N
11	Arthritis	Y/N	Y/N	Y/N

Family history of other diseases:

Relation 1	Illness
Relation 2	Illness
Relation 3	Illness

Personal History
Significant illnesses in the past

Illness 1	Year
Illness 2	Year
Illness 3	Year
Illness 4	Year

Operations:

Type 1	Year
Type 2	Year
Type 3	Year
Type 4	Year

History (before illness started) of:

Asthma	(0–3)	....
Eczema	(0–3)	....
Hayfever	(0–3)	....
Migraine	(0–3)	....
Thyroid disease	Y/N	
Rhinitis	Y/N	
Pernicious anaemia	Y/N	

Do you still suffer from:

Asthma	(0–3)	....
Eczema	(0–3)	....
Hayfever	(0–3)	....
Migraine	(0–3)	....

Thyroid disease   Y/N
Rhinitis   Y/N

History of antibiotics:
How many courses in the last year? ....
How many courses in the previous
four years (approximately)?   ....

History of thrush:
Mouth   Y/N
Bowel   Y/N
Vaginal   Y/N
Anal   Y/N
Penile   Y/N

Drugs:
Has the patient taken any drugs
continuously prior to and since
the onset of this disease process?   Y/N
Name of drug   1
                   2
                   3

History of this current illness
Date of initial onset: Clear/Unclear
History of viral onset: Clear/Unclear

Associated with stress:
Work   Y/N
Occupation   Y/N
Emotional   Y/N
Mental   Y/N
Financial   Y/N
Medical   Y/N
Bereavement   Y/N
Chemical exposure   Y/N
(If yes, give name) ....

Length of illness to date: ....years

Severity of present illness:
Percentage of previous illness

      0–25 per cent
     25–50 per cent
     50–75 per cent
    75–100 per cent

Progress to date:
Improving steadily
Getting steadily worse
Static
Episodic – basically unchanged
Episodic – improving
Episodic – deteriorating
(please encircle relevant progress)

Time after onset of illness for
first consultation with GP ....weeks

Diagnosis at first consultation:
1 Viral – non specific   Y/N
2 Viral – specific (specify)   ....
3 Neurological   Y/N
4 Psychiatric   Y/N
5 Other (specify)   ....

Number of G.P. consultations
before referral: ....
1 Viral – non specific   Y/N
2 Viral – specific (specify)   ....
3 Neurological   Y/N
4 Psychiatric   Y/N
5 Other – (specify)   ....

Time after onset for specialist
consultation ....months

Speciality ....

Diagnosis:
1	Viral – non specific	Y/N
2	Viral – specific(specify)	....
3	Post viral syndrome	Y/N
4	Neurological	Y/N
5	Psychiatric	Y/N
6	Other (specify)	....

How many specialists seen:

	Date	Speciality	Diagnosis
1	.....	....	....
2	.....	....	....
3	.....	....	....
4	.....	....	....
5	.....	....	....
6	.....	....	....
7	.....	....	....
8	.....	....	....
9	.....	....	....
10	.....	....	....

Symptoms:

Major: 1 **Muscular fatigueability** (0–3) .....
             2 **Organic brain effect** (a)
                Concentration loss (0–3) .....
                Loss of thread (0–3) .....
                Unable to finish
                  sentence (0–3) .....
                Unable to follow plot (0–3) .....
                Word difficulty (0–3) .....
                Memory (b)
                Past (0–3) .....
                Recent (0–3) .....

	Retention	(0–3)	

Cognitive problem (c)

	Coordination	(0–3)	.....
	Visuo-spacial	(0–3)	.....
	Clumsy	(0–3)	.....
	Drop things	(0–3)	.....

Mental exhaustion (d)

	Slow thinking	(0–3)	.....

3 Psychiatric

(a)	Emotional	(0–3)	.....
	Mood swings	(0–3)	.....
(b)	Depressed	(0–3)	.....
	Sleep disturbance	(0–3)	.....
	Drive and enthusiasm	(0–3)	.....
(c)	Anxiety:		
	Panic	(0–3)	.....
	Social phobias	(0–3)	.....
	Anxious	(0–3)	.....

Minor:

1 Feeling 'Flu-Like'

Do you feel ill?	(0–3)	.....
Bodily lethargy	(0–3)	.....
Hot/cold	(0–3)	.....
Pyrexia	(0–3)	.....
Aches and pains	(0–3)	.....
Sweating	(0–3)	.....
Sore throats	(0–3)	.....
Cervical glands	(0–3)	.....

2 Central nervous system

Dizziness	(0–3)	.....
Vertigo	(0–3)	.....
Difficulty with eye focusing	(0–3)	.....
Eye pains	(0–3)	.....

Headaches:

	Severity	(0–3)	.....
Frequency:	Constant	Y/N	
	Daily	Y/N	

	Weekly	Y/N
	Monthly	Y/N
Headache exacerbated by physical exertion	(0–3)	.....
Mental stress	(0–3)	.....
Hyperacusis	(0–3)	.....
Nightmares	(0–3)	.....
Pressure (head)	(0–3)	.....

3 Peripheral nervous system
Pins and needles	(0–3)	.....
Burning	(0–3)	.....
Hyperaesthesia	(0–3)	.....
Hypoaesthesia	(0–3)	.....
Numb patches	(0–3)	.....
Shooting nerve pains	(0–3)	.....

4 Musculoskeletal
Muscle stiffness	(0–3)	.....
Muscular weakness	(0–3)	.....
Muscle tenderness	(0–3)	.....
Muscle tender spots	(0–3)	.....
Pain in muscle	(0–3)	.....
Muscle twitching	(0–3)	.....
Bone pains	(0–3)	.....
Joint pains	(0–3)	.....
Joint swelling	(0–3)	.....
Joint stiffness	(0–3)	.....
Small joints	(0–3)	.....
Large joints	(0–3)	.....

5 Cardiovascular system
Peripheral:
Cold hands	(0–3)	.....
Cold feet	(0–3)	.....
Pale colour	(0–3)	.....
Blood drains from face	(0–3)	.....
Chest pains	(0–3)	.....

Short of breath   (0–3)   .....
Palpitations   (0–3)   .....
Purpuric spots   (0–3)   .....
Unexplained bruises   (0–3)   .....

6 Gastro-intestinal system
Indigestion   (0–3)   .....
Nausea   (0–3)   .....
Irritable bowel   (0–3)   .....
Wind   (0–3)   .....
Bloating   (0–3)   .....
Intermittent diarrhoea   (0–3)   .....
Intermittent constipation   (0–3)   .....
Food sensitivity   (0–3)   .....

7 Genito-urinary system
Bladder
    Dysuria   (0–3)   .....
    Urgency   (0–3)   .....
    Frequency   (0–3)   .....
    Incontinence   (0–3)   .....
    Cystitis   (0–3)   .....
Vagina
    Discharge   (0–3)   .....
    Irritation   (0–3)   .....
Penile
    Irritation   (0–3)   .....
    Soreness   (0–3)   .....

8 Specific organ disease viral
Heart myocarditis   Y/N
Pericarditis   Y/N
Encephalitis   Y/N
Meningitis   Y/N
Neuritis   Y/N
Myositis   Y/N
Arthritis   Y/N
Pleurisy   Y/N

Hepatitis   Y/N
Other abdominal viscera   Y/N

9 Environmental symptoms

Food sensitivity

1 Name	(0–3)	.....
2 Name	(0–3)	.....
3 Name	(0–3)	.....
4 Name	(0–3)	.....
5 Name	(0–3)	.....
Multiple others (0–3)	(0–3)	.....

Chemical sensitivity

1 Name	(0–3)	.....
2 Namc	(0–3)	.....
3 Name	(0–3)	.....
4 Name	(0–3)	.....
5 Name	(0–3)	.....

Multiple others (0–3) .....

Drug sensitivity

1 Name	(0–3)	.....
2 Name	(0–3)	.....
3 Name	(0–3)	.....
4 Name	(0–3)	.....
5 Name	(0–3)	.....

Multiple others (0–3) .....

The results

This is the most important section of the book, as it begins to give us an insight into the many factors involved in the development and causative agents of the syndrome, its effects, clinical course, symptomatology and many other aspects.

The questionnaire was filled in for those suffering from AOPVFS, M.E. and for those that did not have M.E. but had been diagnosed as having another disease such as multiple sclerosis. I did not fill in the questionnaire on normal healthy people or those with an acute viral infection as I simply did not have the time; however this ideally needs to be done in order to compare the validity of all of the comments that I have made.

I believe that the questionnaire should also be completed on a number of patients suffering from other chronic disease processes, such as rheumatoid arthritis or multiple sclerosis, to see the presenting features and clinical progress of M.E. and its various types in comparison with other diseases. This is something that we shall clearly have to redress in the near future.

The answers to the questionnaire are now databased and much of the information has yet to be analysed statistically. Where I do have firm answers, suggestions or percentages, I shall state them, and where analysis still has to be done, I shall offer trends that have become apparent.

I shall go through the results in the order that appears on the questionnaire, but some areas are so important that I have expanded on them elsewhere. Where this is the case I shall refer the reader to the relevant pages.

Names, addresses and sex: Some of this is covered in the chapter 'Why ME?' (see p. 186) but what is clearly indicated is that the phenomenon is nation-wide. It showed a large predominance of female sufferers – 78 per cent in the AOPVFS group and 77 per cent in the insidious M.E. group.

Occupation: This showed that a range of socio-economic groups are involved, but the vast majority are mothers who are either housewives primarily or housewives with other jobs, such as nurses, office workers, cleaners, etc. It showed quite clearly that it is not a disease of the upper classes or of hard-working, high-living 'yuppies'.

Work: I was surprised at the morbidity of this disorder. Morbidity is a medical term which refers to the effect that the disease has upon job, life style, etc. and both AOPVFS and M.E. have remarkably similar effects.

Unfortunately, this is one of the areas for which I have not yet been able to get hard figures, but over half of the respondents are severely disabled, and have had to retire medically or have been reduced to part time. This is particularly apparent among the male respondents as it is more pronounced when it affects the primary breadwinner.

The effect on women is much more difficult to see, because they are not usually the primary breadwinner, and therefore giving up their job does not financially affect the family so much as to cause major disruption to the ability to care for home, children and spouse. Most of the women involved had had to give up their occupation where they had one, and then they required a lot of extra help from their husbands, relatives and from statutory bodies in the provision of assistance such as home helps and invalidity benefits.

With regard to children, there were none under the age of seventeen involved in the initial study programme, and my observations on pp. 142–54 are based on those whom I have subsequently studied.

Marital status: I do not yet have the statistical information available, but my observations are that a good few marriages have ended in divorce. This was particularly true in the earlier years of my work in M.E. because the patients' partners were usually told that it was purely psychologically based. They were therefore encouraged to believe that the patient should simply 'pull themselves together' and since this was never achieved, or if so, only very slowly, there were inevitably large areas of friction between the couple.

Fortunately this has changed quite remarkably. Sufferers from AOPVFS or M.E. are now more frequently told what their problem is, so they can accommodate to it and manage their disease; their partner is equally informed, and a much more supportive bond tends to develop. The separation and divorce rate has fallen quite dramatically in the last year or so. This must be considered as being one of the important effects of widespread publicity and understanding.

General observations also tell me that the vast majority (probably 90 per cent) are married, and 80 per cent or so of those are female; the vast majority have children.

Family history: There were only four people in whom at least one other member of the family was believed to suffer from the same phenomenon. My further studies continue to demonstrate that the vast majority of disease is seen in single cases, sporadically presented with no obvious connection with any other member of the family or of the community.

Family history(2): There did not appear to be any relationship of this disease to a family history of any of the eleven disorders mentioned here.

Family history of any other disease: So far there does not appear to be any significant relationship between AOPVFS and the family history of any other disease process.

Personal history: The very definition of AOPVFS does not allow for any significant illness to have been experienced that could in any way contribute to the current symptomatology. Therefore there must necessarily be medical exclusions in this category, and whether in future one will be able to tie up any other significant illnesses experiencèd in the past with the development of M.E. and its various subsets remains to be seen. Again by definition, any illnesses that had been experienced were trivial, and a full recovery had been made.

History of other associated disorders: The figures here initially seemed to be quite high. Asthma, eczema and hayfever were present in 34 per cent of AOPVFS and 38 per cent of M.E. sufferers but the same very high figures were found in the control group. It just goes to show how common they are.

In any event, there was no statistical association between the development of disease and a predisposing 'allergic' type background. The same was applicable to thyroid disorder, rhinitis or pernicious anaemia, which might have otherwise suggested a possible auto immune predisposition. A brief explanation of auto immune disorder follows.

Quite frequently, especially with increasing age, the body unfortunately develops the capability of attacking itself. The immune system evolves an abnormal immunological response and produces antibodies to one's own tissue. The body no longer recognizes parts of itself as being itself, this self-attacking immunological response slowly destroys the tissues involved and disease appears. Examples of such disease processes include rheumatoid arthritis, an arterial disease called polyarteritis nodosum, and myasthenia gravis (a muscle wasting disease).

I mention this auto immune disorder because after the onset of AOPVFS a few patients were observed to develop an auto immune thyroid disorder. This came to light when considering the next question, **Do you still suffer from**?, where seven patients had difficulty in answering the question on thyroid disease. They had not had thyroid disease before, but had afterwards developed a virus type of thyroid inflammation called Hashimoto's thyroiditis, named after a Japanese physician, Dr Hashimoto.

With regard to the other questions in this section, where the patients had been observed to have asthma, eczema, hayfever, migraine, thyroid disease or rhinitis prior to AOPVFS or M.E. they continued still to suffer from that.

One question of course which was not applicable to the AOPVFS group was that of thyroid disease, because if they had had it prior to their disease development they would have automatically been excluded from the study.

History of antibiotics: This question was put in mainly to see if there was any relationship between excessive exposure to antibiotics and the development of either M.E. or AOPVFS. We found that, on average, only one course of antibiotics had been taken in the year prior to the development of either M.E. or AOPVFS and statistically there was no inclination to that course of antibiotics immediately preceding the illness.

The questionnaire has only been completed by the initial patients, and I have no further information on this as regards the subsequent patients I have investigated – so one could argue that this study represents quite a small number and may not be statistically significant. However, as on average only four courses of antibiotics were given in the previous four years, there did not appear to be any chronic excessive ingestion of antibiotics.

There are a great number of people who believe that M.E. is directly related to the excessive intake of antibiotics and the subsequent development of candida albicans (thrush). Again, there were no particular observations to be made when looking at the history of thrush. Only one female respondent had mouth thrush in the preceding year, and nobody offered a history of bowel, anal or penile thrush. Vaginal thrush showed a 10 per cent positive response, a figure reflected in the normal population, so there does not appear to be any link between thrush, antibiotics and the development of the disease. Whether or not candida albicans has a part to play in the subsequent symptomatology is explored in pp. 236–39.

Drugs: AOPVFS did not show anybody taking a medication on a continuous basis. In the M.E. group, 10 per cent were intermittently taking painkillers in the form of aspirin, paracetamol, or ibuprofen for their headaches, but it was as a consequence of the disorder, rather than a predisposing contributing factor.

History of this current illness: The two questions here gave us the ability to differentiate between AOPVFS and slower onset M.E., because if the patient could remember the actual date that the illness started it was deemed to be an acute onset. The way in which that was assessed was along the following lines.

As some patients with this disorder had had it for a considerable length of time before the interview (approximately two years) they had sometimes forgotten the date that it all started. They would initially say, for example, that it probably began in spring two years ago. I would then start to narrow this down by asking questions like 'Was this immediately before Easter or after Easter?' We could then track it down to a few days of a particular month with some degree of certainty. Then I would ask them whether there was a particular day in which they became unwell, when the day prior to that they would have described themselves as being fit and normal.

The acute onset type always fitted into this pattern. Sixty per cent also spontaneously included a comment such as 'Yes – I was absolutely fit, but I was certainly more tired than usual for about a week or a fortnight before this started.' 'I did not have any symptoms, but I felt a little run down, and then I came home from work because I developed this typical flu-like illness.'

I always spent a great deal of time on this particular part of the story, as it is extremely important to be able to pinpoint a day. To take the patients back a couple of years or so to how they felt that day was often difficult, but usually very rewarding. They started to relive that day which, while initially thought to be forgotten, was clearly a major event in their lives, and probably not pushed very far into the subconscious.

To actually establish whether this was a 'virus' at the beginning was again difficult, but to be able to decide whether it was an upper respiratory tract infection was not particularly hard; they would usually say, 'I had a sore throat, aches and pains, and a temperature with a headache', and so on. Some did not have a sore throat, and that made it a little more of a problem, but a typical viral story would be that of an acute malaise, headaches, widespread aches and pains, feeling hot and cold, and a raised temperature.

Association with stress: This is dealt with on pp. 132–33 in full detail, but in general terms this series of questions was put in because I had noticed how many people had spontaneously said that they were under a great deal of stress – that they were working hard, there were problems at home or within the marriage, or they were under general strain. It was very common to find that young women, being both mothers and working outside the home, found a great deal of pressure in trying to cope with all of the things that they were required to do.

Stress frequently expressed itself in the development of psychological symptoms such as anxiety, depression and sleep disturbance, and also physical symptoms – coming home from work feeling exhausted, needing to go to bed earlier than usual.

The individual figures have not yet been analysed, but a total figure of 86 per cent of AOPVFS patients suggested stress as a contributing factor. The degree of stress involved in the development of M.E. was impossible to assess, because if the disease is insidious, with no obvious starting point, then the amount of stress required to contribute to that has to be over a longer period of time than that seen in AOPVFS.

The stress of bereavement had not occurred in any AOPVFS respondents nor was there any involvement with chemical exposure.

The length of the illness to date: The average length of illness was one and a half years, and none of the patients had been ill less than one year.

Severity of present illness: This was taken in conjunction with progress to date. There are, however, no markers for this disorder, as there are no specific tests to show the degree of intensity of M.E., so I had to measure their illness in overall functional capability. The concepts of being 25–50 or 75 per cent ill were arbitrary, and I decided that I would have to draw a graph of their disease process measuring 'subjective illness' for each of the patients I interviewed (see pp. 161 and 180). The graph was then viewed in conjunction with the questionnaire, allowing a much more detailed analysis of the progress of the disorder.

The answers to the questions: Time after onset of illness for first consultation with GP; Diagnosis on first consultation; Number of GP consultations before referral; Time after onset for specialist consultation; Diagnosis; and How many specialists seen? have not yet been fully analysed. However, my estimate is that the AOPVFS patients visited their GP within the first week of the disease, and that the initial diagnosis was a non-specific viral infection in some 80 per cent or so of cases.

The number of subsequent consultations with the GP about the same complaint was high – probably around five consultations before referral to hospital. In approximately 50 per cent of cases the initial specialist diagnosis was also a non-specific viral infection, but continuing referral for further advice tended to lead to a psychiatric diagnosis – in other words, while AOPVFS patients are told they have a virus infection at the beginning of their disease, when the expected recovery does not occur the diagnosis changes. After a year and a half, 90 per cent of patients are told that they do not have anything wrong with them, that their problem is stress-related, or that they are overtly suffering from a psychiatric illness.

In slow onset M.E. the number obtaining an initial physical diagnosis was much lower, and the length of time taken to present to their GP with the non-specific symptomatology was much longer – somewhere between three to six months. The initial diagnosis was either psychiatric or something such as anaemia, hormonal change, debility, age etc. The number of GP consultations in this group was also higher than in the AOPVFS group, being in excess of ten before a hospital referral. Once a consultant opinion was sought, the number obtaining a physical diagnosis of any kind was very low – 10 per cent or less. It was much more common in this group to find a psychiatric consultant opinion being sought initially, and the resulting psychiatric diagnosis was much higher – 70 per cent or more.

Subsequent to this questionnaire the picture has slightly altered. Many more doctors are now prepared to make a diagnosis of post viral syndrome, and I believe that this reflects the change of medical opinion in this field. However, while doctors are more ready to diagnose post viral syndrome, whether they believe it to be physically or psychologically based is still a thorny problem. I feel that somewhere in the region of 50 per cent of GPs and consultants are still of the opinion that post viral syndrome is a psychiatric process.

Symptoms: The symptoms are given here in absolute percentage terms. I have not been able to analyse the degree of the symptom complained of, as measured by a reply from the patient of 0, 1, 2 or 3. Again, there is a lack of control material, in that I did not interview normal patients or those with other diseases to see if the symptoms were apparent there.

Symptom	AOPVFS %	M.E. %	NOT M.E. %
Muscular fatigueability	[100]	[98]	[34]
Organic brain effect:			
Concentration	82	74	60
Thread	70	75	72
Sentence	61	68	59
Plot	50	63	54
Word	74	67	not done
Memory:			
Past	4	7	[20]
Recent	[92]	[84]	38
Retention	[94]	[84]	58

Cognitive problem:

Coordination	15	12	17
Visuo-spacial	21	11	11
Clumsy	18	12	12
Drop things	21	12	16

Mental exhaustion:

Slow thinking	76	62	64

Psychiatric:

Emotional	[83]	40	15
Mood swings	[76]	39	18
Depressed	71	68	79
Sleep disturbance	[63]	40	33
Drive and enthusiasm	70	49	80

Anxiety:

Panic	40	32	21
Social phobias	[42]	30	15
Anxious	[69]	31	22

Feeling 'flu-like':	[84]	73	41
Bodily lethargy	88	80	74
Hot cold	[62]	42	22
Pyrexia	2	4	8
Aches and pains	[79]	[83]	31
Sweating	[54]	[43]	9
Sore throat	[33]	[44]	10
Glands	[29]	[15]	3

Central nervous system:

Dizziness	72	70	79
Vertigo	15	27	28
Focusing	[58]	[47]	16
Eye pains	4	15	29
Headache	[90]	[92]	[88]

Severity **	–	–	–
Constant **	–	–	–

Daily **	–	–	–
Weekly **	–	–	–
Monthly **	–	–	–
Headache:			
Physical exertion **	–	–	–
Mental stress **			
Hyperacusis **	–	–	–
Nightmares	24	39	15
Head pressure	62	41	59
Peripheral nervous system:			
Pins and needles *			
Durning *			
Hyperaesthesia *			
Hypoaesthesia *			
Numb patches *			
Shooting nerve pains *			
	74*	82*	91*
Musculoskeletal:			
Muscle stiffness	40	63	58
Muscle weakness	[91]	[75]	[88]
Muscle tenderness	59	62	32
Muscle tender spots	[63]	[71]	[50]
Muscle pain	[80]	[74]	34
Muscle twitching	63	64	51
Bone pain			
Joint pain	17	29	25
Joint swelling	2	5	15
Joint stiffness			
Small joints	8	18	23
Large joints			
Cardiovascular system:			
Cold hands			
Cold feet	[73]	[69]	11
Pale colour	[66]	[57]	18

Blood drains	[61]	[48]	12
Chest pains	69	58	50
Short of breath	[42]	21	19
Palpitations	39	28	33
Purpuric spots	0	2	4
Bruises	5	8	20

Gastro-intestinal system:
Indigestion *
Nausea *
Irritable bowel *
Wind *
Bloating *
Intermittent diarrhoea*
Constipation *

	[24]*	[26]*	6*
Food sensitivity	[18]	[24]	6

Genito–urinary system:
Bladder:

Dysuria	2	1	1
Urgency	4	7	3
Frequency	15	7	6
Incontinence	0	0	1
Cystitis	10	8	8

Vagina:

Discharge	9	5	3
Irritation	8	7	4

Penis:

Irritation	0	0	1
Soreness	0	0	1

Specific organ disease viral:
Myocarditis

Pericarditis	[7]	2	0
Encephalitis			
Meningitis	[3]	0	0

Neuritis	0	0	0
Myositis	0	0	0
Arthritis	0	0	0
Pleurisy	2	0	0
Hepatitis	1	0	0
Other	–	–	–

Environmental symptoms:

Food sensitivity	Not suitable for analysis
Chemical sensitivity	Not suitable for analysis
Drug sensitivity	Not suitable for analysis

[ ] denotes figures of particular statistical significance

*Overall %

**Figures not yet available

I do not think it appropriate to discuss in detail all the symptoms and their possible interpretation. However, it is evident that there are areas of symptomatology which are common to AOPVFS and M.E. in a significantly higher level than is found in the group not suffering from either disease. One can also see some symptoms that appear to be more prevalent in AOPVFS than in the slow onset group; these on the whole tend to be the acute type, such as feeling ill, with hot and cold sweats.

Some of the psychiatric symptomatology is also more prevalent in the AOPVFS group, emotional lability and sleep disturbance being particularly noticeable. One can see that there are groups of symptoms associated with both disorders, muscle fatigue of course being an essential finding, memory problems being almost exclusively confined to recent memory and to memory retention.

Flu-like symptoms are also predominant, the general concept of feeling ill, with aches, pains and sweats and sore glands and throat occurring on average in over 50 per cent of sufferers. The occurrence of headache does not seem to be greater than is seen in non M.E. groups, but the difficulty in focusing referred to as accommodation is quite pronounced.

Muscular symptoms are again predominant. One comment I would make here is that muscular weakness is a subjective feeling; on examination there is very little in the way of a demonstrable weakening of muscle capability. However, muscle pain, discomfort and tender spots are very high in both groups of disease, but this is also the case in the non M.E. group.

Cardiovascular symptoms are clearly pronounced in the disease group, as against the non M.E. group, with a high instance of cold hands and feet, pallor and draining of facial colour.

Apart from these quite clear trends, one must comment on the fact that all three groups are polysymptomatic. They have a great number of symptoms and they appear to occur at quite intense levels, and this is something that requires further investigation.

Genito-urinary symptoms are very low, and there does not appear to be a significantly high level of symptomatology that might indicate any specific involvement with candida albicans. Unfortunately, the food, drug and chemical sensitivity answers have not at present been found suitable for analysis.

It should be noted that 7 per cent of AOPVFS and 3 per cent of M.E. cases appear to be associated with pericomyocarditis – a viral infection of the lining of the heart and of the heart muscle. This disease has long been associated with the enteroviruses and, apart from encephalitis and meningitis constituting 3 per cent, is the only significant organ inflammatory process noted at the beginning of the disease.

5

IMMUNOLOGY

The whole concept of M.E. seems to revolve around predisposing factors, viruses, and immunology. We talk about environmental factors, drugs, antibiotics, chemicals that suppress the immune system, abnormal immunological responses, specific immunocompromisation and the like.

The immune system is a vast and complex interaction of various white cell functions. These cells are made in different parts of the body – bone marrow, spleen etc. – and are closely interactive, being stimulated or suppressed by chemicals secreted by themselves, so that they can communicate with each other. They act as a vigilant guard, and when presented with foreign bodies in the form of chemicals, toxins, proteins, bacteria, viruses etc. set up a chain of events which hopefully results in the elimination of the invader. In order to survive, the body has developed a complex series of systems to defend itself against these 'antigens'.

An antigen is any substance which, when it enters the body, is recognized by the immune system as being foreign. Antigens are usually complex molecules, and consist of sugars, amino acids or lipids. They come in many shapes and many sizes. For example, the enterovirus antigen, which is referred to as virus protein 1, is an amino acid chain called a polypeptide and many of these constitute a protein. This is recognized by the immune system as being antigenic and the body will make an appropriate antibody to it.

Antigens come up against a first line of defence called a natural or innate immunity. If this immunity is overcome the whole of the

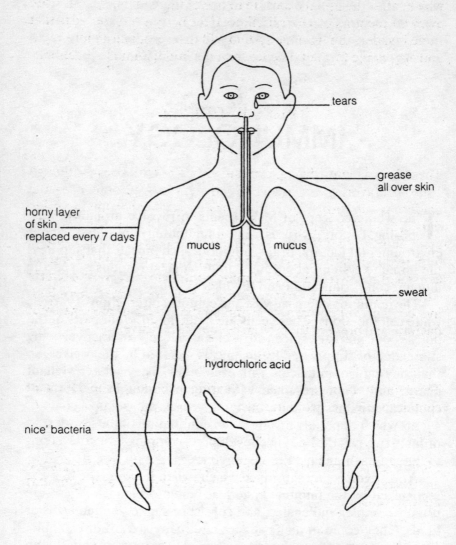

Fig. 1 The physical and chemical barriers of natural immunity

immune system comes into play and is responsible for the immune reaction and the production of the state of acquired immunity which, after the initial exposure to one of these invaders, can store away the memory of it for a lifetime. If the body is re-exposed to that same invader, the immune system will then produce a more rapid and aggressive form of defence than the initial immune reaction.

Innate immunity

The skin

The skin is a highly dynamic organ, varying in thickness, although 1mm is the average. It has several active layers. The outer one – the epidermis – is constantly being renewed, growing from the inside outwards, and has a turnover of some seven days. As the cells grow outward they dry up, so the outermost layer is a thick, scaly, impervious protective membrane which can repair wounds and act as a shield against the many different types of chemicals and bacteria – the 'flora' – resident on the skin. They are usually quite harmless, indeed, their very presence can inhibit the growth of more harmful bacteria and prevent them from becoming invasive.

Sweat

This liquid is being produced at varying levels all of the time, and contains antibacterial chemicals.

Grease

More correctly referred to as sebum, it is constantly being made and secreted from specific little glands in the skin and again has antimicrobial effects.

Tears and mucus

Rather like sweat, tears contain antibacterial and antiviral substances, specifically lysozymes. The latter can also be found in mucus secreted from the nose, mouth, lung and vagina (the vagina also secretes very acid mucus which in itself is inhibitory to bacteria).

The gastro-intestinal system

This kills viruses and bacteria with acidic mucus from the stomach and inhibitory bacteria present in normal gut. For instance, there are enormous numbers of flora which are resident in the bowel, mainly bacteria like E. coli, which are not only necessary for normal bowel function, digestion and vitamin absorption but also inhibit the growth of harmful bacteria. The mucus secreted from the gastro-intestinal system also contains specific antibody.

Thus you can see that there is a widespread initial defence system. It is rather like a perimeter fence with barbed wire, a general protector to keep invaders out. These innate defence systems cannot be mustered into action and they do not occur in very high levels, so it is relatively easy to lower their effectiveness – for example, the harmless bacteria found on the skin should not be too frequently scrubbed off, as a much more aggressive bug such as Stap. Aureous can get into the skin follicle and cause carbuncles or abcesses. Upsetting the gastro-intestinal flora by taking too many antibiotics can kill off the harmless E. coli, thus leading to an overgrowth of yeasts such as candida albicans which causes thrush in the mouth and the vagina, or can allow the gastro-intestinal tract to be overrun by other bacteria which upset the digestive system, giving rise to colitis or irritable bowel syndrome. The same sort of phenomenon is seen in women who take the oral contraceptive pill, which can allow the development of some candidal infection, usually within the vagina and arguably in the gut.

There are those who suggest that toxic chemicals can disturb this gastro-intestinal balance and can be predisposing to various disease processes, including some fatigue syndromes. I am not at all sure about this myself and I do not at present advocate that interpretation; this whole field of medicine is a controversial one, to say the least.

Acquired or active Immunity

Let us assume now that the antigen has broken through this passive barrier and entered the body via some kind of damage. It will find that there is again a non-specific defence system, but this time it is much more active and aggressive. These antigens, be they poisons such as a bee sting, food bacteria, viruses or whatever will be faced with various enzymes, complement (the immunological enzymes system), lysozymes, acute phase proteins, and other very complex chemicals which are produced by an increase of blood flow to the damaged area, and a stimulation and mustering of white cell defence. These antigens can then be directly 'eaten' by specifically designed white cells called macrophages and by polymorphonuclear cells which generally wander around the tissues in and outside the bloodstream looking for aggressive and noxious agents. Invading antigens absorbed into the system are filtered out by lymph nodes which contain tens of millions of active white cells, specifically designed for the purpose; harmful chemicals can be detoxified.

At the time of conception, we are supplied with genetic coding material which enables us to recognize several million substances or antigens as being foreign and harmful, and we are endowed with the capability of developing a very complicated series of systems and reactions to make a specific antibody to each antigen. The antibody attacks and neutralizes the antigen and this antibody antigen complex is subsequently removed and rendered harmless.

Antibodies are chemicals that are produced by B-cell lymphocytes. They are developed to be highly specific, and are directed to combine with, and assist in the neutralization of, antigens.

An antibody is a protein and there are several of them, collectively referred to as immunoglobulins. Because of their various shapes and sizes they can be sub-divided into classes or groups (see Fig.2)

It can be seen that they all have a 'Y' shape. The highly active end, and the bit that we really want to look at, is the combining site.

It is this portion of the immunoglobulin that is very critical in its shape and its build-up, as this area defines the response of that antibody in combining with its specific antigen. Each IgG produced is the long-term antibody to a specific antigen. For example, if you are stung by a wasp, the venom injected will stimulate your immune system to make an antibody to it. That antibody will attack wasp's venom, but it will not attack mosquito venom, or bee sting, or snake bite, or

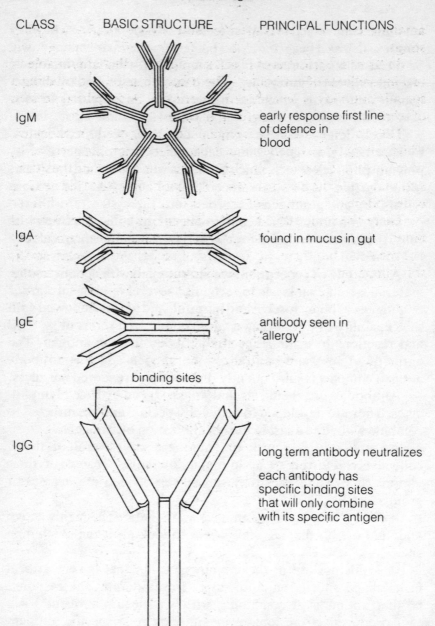

CLASS   BASIC STRUCTURE   PRINCIPAL FUNCTIONS

IgM — early response first line of defence in blood

IgA — found in mucus in gut

IgE — antibody seen in 'allergy'

binding sites

IgG — long term antibody neutralizes

each antibody has specific binding sites that will only combine with its specific antigen

Fig. 2 Structure and shape of the various antibodies found in the blood

anything else. It is the specific antibody developed for wasp stings.

So there are millions of B-cell's in the body that are capable of making millions of antibodies. The B-cell's capability of making a specific antibody is determined genetically. A simplified version of what happens goes something like this:

There are specific antigen recognizing cells called lymphocytes, which are found inside the bloodstream. Blood consists of red cells, which give it its colour, platelets, which are used in coagulation, and various white cells; the rest, probably about 45 per cent, is called plasma.

There are some 100,000 white cells in one cubic centimetre of blood, i.e., there are some 5,000,000 in the bloodstream at any one moment, but there are also tens of millions localized in small, soft lymph nodules scattered around the body. Lymphocytes are

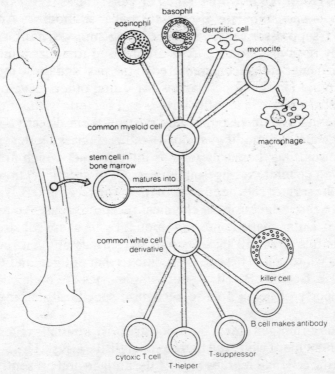

Fig. 3   How the various white blood cells develop

also found in the spleen and in the bone marrow, where they are actually made.

Lymphocytes start off life as a stem cell in the bone marrow; they then divide and produce many sorts of lymphocytes (see Fig.3). Some travel through the blood to the thymus gland, which is situated in the upper front part of the chest, and here a complex reaction occurs; the cells are modified, and they become what are known as thymic lymphocytes (T-cells). These T-cells have specific functions, especially that of the recognition of specific antigens, and they also develop the power of control over other lymphocytes, i.e. those that do not pass through the thymus gland and are found in the spleen and the lymph glands – the B-lymphocytes. These specific B-lymphocytes have the task of developing and making specific antibodies.

There are many, many different types of T-cells, and here I will discuss just some of their functions.

One group is known as T-helper cells; these travel through the blood and stimulate B-cells to make antibodies. Another group, T-suppressor cells, will come along and switch off a B-cell antibody response. Some T-cells are devised to act as a memory for a particular antigen encountered in the past and these memory cells can hide in the bone marrow for years; others develop into killer cells, which can identify viruses and bacteria without the aid of any other system response and destroy them directly. T-cells also regulate and modify various B-cell responses by developing and transmitting chemicals such as interleukines which are used to pass on general messages and messages of specific action.

On the surface cell membrane of these various T and B-lymphocytes are three-dimensional chemical receptor areas. An antigen has a particular shape conferred upon it by its chemical structure and it is this structure that fits into the surface antigen receptor site of a white cell. This site is specific to that antigen and to that particular T-cell or B-cell, so our lymphocytes are endowed with the property of being able to recognize specifically an invading antigen.

When an antigen enters the bloodstream it is initially recognized by another type of white cell that has many little 'arms'. This is called a dendritic cell, and it grabs hold of the antigen and presents it to a T-helper cell, whereupon the antigen is then presented to the B-cell specific to it. The helper cells stimulate the B-cells to divide and to produce many daughter cells, and to make a specific antibody to that antigen. The antibody latches on to the antigen and neutralizes it, and then this antigen antibody complex is cleared from the system by white cells called macrophages.

In the early stage of this antibody production the class of antibody produced is an IgM antibody. Later, the longer term neutralizing IgG antibody is produced and it is at this stage that the antigen has been got under control. The T-suppressor cell will then develop a switch-off response to the B-cell, the IgM response will begin to disappear and the IgG response will lessen, and the whole system begins to settle down. As the antigen disappears from the body, a few T-cells will hide away to produce a memory response, and a few B cells will also remain dormant in the lympathic systems. This allows the body to make a much more vigorous and amplified response should that antigen ever be encountered again. The memory cell will recognize the antigen and switch on the memory B-cells rapidly, and a much more effective and early antibody response will be found. The antigen will therefore be eradicated sooner and more devastatingly.

This gives a small insight into the body's immunological defence systems, but as we have a specific interest in viruses, I will discuss a few extra cards that the immunological response has to offer. When viruses enter the body, they have to multiply inside cells – for example, if an infected person coughs over you, you will then inhale infected virus droplets into the nose or the mouth. Here they enter by penetrating the mucous membranes at the back of the throat and from there they successfully evade your innate or natural immune system to a greater or lesser extent. Once inside these cells in the throat the virus will multiply and, when filled with new virus, the cell will burst open and the newly made virus will sweep into the bloodstream and invade other body cells, for example in the brain or the muscles. By this time you are well into your 'flu'.

The body's more active defence mechanism will try to eat up the virus directly with white cells (macrophages). It will also switch on B-cells (antibodies) which attack the virus particles in the bloodstream but, so far, there is nothing to stop the virus inside the cells of the muscle or the brain. Once those viruses are in there, it seems that they will evade the body's immune defence mechanisms.

Chemicals such as interferon can be produced to counter the viruses. This substance lines the membrane of the cells of the body generally and prevents further spread of the virus and penetration of that virus into the cell. Interferon also produces a lot of the symptoms of flu – the malaise, the aches and pains, the temperature etc.

There are also further attacking moves that the immune system has developed, and one of these is the specific T-killer cell. Once a virus enters a cell, it leaves a mark on the surface. A T-killer cell can recognize the marks on the surface and, by attaching itself to the membrane of that virus infected cell, can literally open it up, and kill the virus inside.

The body's defences consist of these and many more intricate processes, finely balanced and highly tuned cellular reactions that produce specific antibodies and other chemicals that will neutralize invading antigen. These thousands of reactions, most of which I have not even touched upon, require hundreds of chemicals and it can be easily appreciated that the immune system is a highly complex and delicate mechanism.

6

VIROLOGY

The subject of virology is an enormous field, and extremely complex, so I am going to keep it reasonably simple and discuss it in basic terms, specifically in its relationship to M.E. Consequently, I shall describe the enteroviruses and the Epstein Barr virus (EBV).

What is a virus?

A virus is the smallest particle currently known that is capable of causing an infection and a disease process. There are thousands of different viruses, and those under discussion here should be imagined as being rather like a table tennis ball with a pea inside it. The table tennis ball has an irregular surface and is called a capsule; the central pea is referred to as the nucleus or genome.

When looking at EBV, there are sometimes other layers around the outer aspect of the capsule which are important. If you take a virus out of context and simply put it under the microscope, it can be seen to be made up variably of lipid (bits of fat), carbohydrate (bits of starch) and amino acids or nucleic bases (protein). These organic chemicals and substances are arranged in a very complex way so as to make every virus specific, which allows their identification and classification.

The arrangements of these compounds on the surface and the outermost parts of the virus allow that virus to have a very specific capability of attaching itself to complementary structures inside the human body – in other words, they have predefined three-dimensionally arranged probes, which will fit into an equal configuration on the surface of the cell, called a receptor site. This allows that particular virus to attach itself to that particular cell, and none other. This is the reason why, say, the common cold virus will attack the lining of your nose and give you a specific set of symptoms, but will not affect a cat, which does not have that particular receptor site.

A virus on the table is an inert structure; it is lifeless, it does not breathe, it does not feed, it cannot reproduce; it is just an arrangement of chemical compounds. It is a parasite and a passive invader, so how does a virus cause your particular disease?

How does a virus infect?

There are many ways in which viruses can enter the body, but the viruses in question here accomplish it in two ways – through the nose and through the mouth.

Once the infecting virus has entered the body, it attaches itself to the membrane wall of the host cell, using its specific matching receptor site. Processes then occur that allow the viral genome to breach the cell membrane, and it then goes inside the cell with its nuclear material to start its replicating process.

The viral genetic material is either ribonucleic acid (RNA) or deoxyribonucleic (DNA) and consists of nucleic bases (organic molecules) arranged in various sequences. These sequences are called genes, and they consist of codes. This genetic material takes over the cell in a variety of ways but, basically, once a virus is inside the cell it takes over the whole cellular function, and converts that cell into a virus producing factory. In this way, the encoded messages in the viral genetic material cause the cell to make virus proteins, virus capsules, more virus genome etc. Once the capsule and the genome have been made the genome is put into the capsule and the cell is filled with virus.

By now, the cell is usually doomed. The membrane bursts, and hundreds of new infective virus particles are spilled out into the various body systems. So the virus spreads, possibly to the next door cell, but also through the lymphatic system and the bloodstream, where they flow with the circulation and rapidly reach all parts of the body. Which cell is infected next depends upon the receptor site – if the cell receptor site is correct, then the virus will penetrate that cell.

For instance, Coxsackie B has a high affinity for going into muscle, but may not affect white cells or other non-specific cell tissue, whereas Epstein Barr virus has an affinity for attacking particular white cells, but no mechanism for going into muscle. So you can see how a particular virus will give you specific symptoms, as well as the more general ones.

After the initial penetration of a virus into a cell there is a variable period of incubation. This can be as little as two or three days, as in the common cold, or as long as several months, as in rabies. Once the virus starts to spill into the bloodstream or the lymphatic system, and starts a generalized spread, it is accompanied by the clinical phenomenon known as the prodromal phase. This occurs before the full-blown infection becomes apparent, and gives rise to that feeling of 'I think that I am going to go down with something'.

The prodromal phase symptoms found in the initial phase of most virus infections are a low grade fever, feeling unwell, perhaps a headache, aches and pains, etc. This phase of rapid virus spread and uptake into other cells is accompanied by the body's initial immune response.

At the beginning, the response is rather non-specific, and such substances as interferon are produced. This chemical can prevent the virus going into other cells and thus limits the infection, but its very production causes the aches and pains, the headache, the malaise, hot and cold sweats etc. So it is the body's defence mechanism that produces the symptoms of flu – not the virus itself, but the body's response to it.

There are many other complex reactions which follow in a chain of events, brought about by the mobilization of the body's specific immune defence mechanisms, which, by now, are beginning to swing into action.

Once a virus has entered a cell, it leaves a mark on the surface. That surface marker has at least two functions: one is that it prevents penetration of more virus into that cell; the second is that it allows specific white cells to identify that cell, whereupon they will attack and kill the cell and the infective virus being made inside. Other white cells now develop activity.

The white cells known as B-lymphocytes and T-lymphocytes have a complex interaction; they recognize viruses in the bloodstream or elsewhere and kill them directly, or the B-lymphocytes can be switched on to make antibody under the control of many factors. The antibody so produced is specifically directed towards the virus; it attaches itself to the virus particle and begins to neutralize it to prevent it from becoming continuously infective. This neutralized antibody/virus couple is called an immune complex.

These complexes can then be cleared away by other white cells called macrophages, which eat up neutralized virus. At the time of this sequence of events, the patient is just about at the height of his or her infection, probably lying in bed feeling at death's door! He or she is also at his or her most infectious phase. There will be a lot of virus about, probably being secreted by a cough in droplets that float in the atmosphere, ready to infect another person. Alternatively, the virus may be thrown out in large quantities in the stool.

Hopefully a turn for the better now occurs. Antibodies are being made in profusion, activated white cells are munching up more virus than can be produced, and the whole immunological process of response is getting the upper hand. Interferon production ceases, the aches and pains, malaise and fever disappear, and the patient, though battle-scarred, weak and fatigued, becomes less infectious, begins his or her recovery phase and, in the normal course of events, regains strength. The white cell response begins to diminish, the numbers of white cells subside, but the body will remember this infection, hopefully, for a lifetime, as some very specific white cells disappear into the bone marrow or hide away in lymph glands, carrying with them a specific coding of 'memory' within their structure. These ensure that if the same virus comes along again, the immunological response can be that much more aggressive and rapidly mobilized.

Most viruses cause this type of memory response and, provided the virus does not change its shape or its coding, you will not get that virus more than once, unless there is a specific immunological problem that could upset that memory response. There are, however, a number of viruses which are capable of rapid change –

notoriously the cold and influenza viruses, which can alter their shape just enough to prevent the body being able to recognize them immediately. That is why you can get one cold after another, throughout your life.

It is worth examining in more detail the viruses that are of concern to M.E. sufferers – the group of enteroviruses and the Epstein Barr virus.

Picorna viridae

The name picorna virus was initially introduced in general virological terms in 1963. It was developed in order to include not only the enteroviruses, but also the rhinoviruses.

Two of the properties of the various viruses and their subgroups are that there are not affected when you try to dissolve them in ether, and that the centre of the virus, the genome, is made of RNA. The name picorna was derived from an acronym, thus: P (polio virus); I (insensitivity to ether); C (Coxsackie virus); O (orphan virus); R (rhinovirus); R (ribo); N (nucleic); A (acid). One of the two Rs then disappeared and a double-barrelled name PICO-RNA was developed because of another character of these viruses; pico means very small, and certainly the RNA viruses are so.

After 1963, various classification techniques were adopted to find out which viruses constituted this group, taking both their physical and biochemical characteristics into account. The officially accepted group name of picorna viridae was developed by Melmick in 1974, and there are four groups of viruses within it: 1) The enteroviruses; 2) The cardioviruses; 3) The rhinoviruses; 4) The aphthoviruses.

The enteroviruses

The virus is symmetrical particle which has a diameter of 27 nanometers, that is, 1 metre $\times$ 10^{-9}. (0.0000000001 metres). It is one of the smallest viruses known. It consists of a capsule, or capsid, with a genome inside. The capsid is made purely of polypeptides, a series of amino acids arranged in long chains. It does not contain any lipid or carbohydrate.

The virus capsule is an icosahedron – that is to say it has twenty sides. Each of these twenty sides is the same shape, and is made of four major proteins of different shapes and sizes.

One molecule of each of these four proteins makes up one surface and by their spatial arrangement some sixty of these molecules make up the surface of the shell. The four proteins are called VP1, VP2, VP3 and VP4 respectively (VP stands for virus protein). The shell itself is about 2 nanogrammes in thickness and inside it lies the virus genome. This is a single strand of ribonucleic acid (RNA) which consists of approximately 30 per cent of the protein weight of the virus molecule. RNA is made of nucleic acid bases, and there are four of these bases arranged in various sequences which determine the genetic messages and tell the infected cell exactly what action to take when the virus invades.

The RNA itself is the infectious portion of the virus. Virus multiplication occurs in the cytoplasm of the infected cell, and once the RNA has taken over the cell's production it simply reproduces one long duplicate chain of proteins and nucleic bases which are then broken up by specifically produced enzymes. All of the small virus proteins that are thus made form new virus particles.

The enteroviruses can be denatured by relatively mild conditions. For instance, a little bit of ultra-violet light destroys them, and so does heating them for about ten minutes at 56°C. However, they are very resistant to acid and can withstand brief exposure to a Ph of 2. They can thus pass readily through the stomach, where the hydrochloric acid destroys and denatures most viruses.

The enteroviruses are divided into five groups: polio; Coxsackie group A; Coxsackie B; ECHO (enteropathogenic cytopathogenic human orphan) virus; and human enteroviruses.

The polio viruses were first identified in 1909. Later, in 1948, Dalldorf and Sickles discovered a new group of viruses by chance. Until that time the only way of isolating the polio virus was to grow it in monkeys. Because they had to be destroyed to find the virus this was a very expensive method and was not considered to be a good way of diagnosing the problem.

Types of human enteroviruses

Group	Virus types/Major disease associations
Poliovirus	3 types (poliovirus 1–3) Paralytic poliomyelitis – aseptic meningitis
Coxsackievirus Group A	23types (A1-A22-A24) Aseptic meningitis – herpangina – acute febrile illness – conjunctivitis [A24]
Coxsackievirus Group B	6 types (B1-B6) Aseptic meningitis – severe generalized neonatal disease – myocarditis – encephalitis – pleurodynia (Bornholm disease)
Echovirus	31 types (1–9, 11–27, 29–33) Aseptic meningitis with or without rash – febrile disease – conjunctivitis
Enteroviruses	5 types (68–72) Polio-like illness (E71) – pandemic conjunctivitis (E70) – Hepatitis A (E72)

So Dalldorf and Sickles were looking for a new laboratory animal to use, and it was while they were working on newborn mice and studying some faecal extracts from two children who had a paralytic type of disease that they discovered the new non-polio type viruses. These were named Coxsackie viruses, because the two children in whom they were discovered came from a town in New York State called Coxsackie.

Many new viruses then became apparent, and they were sub-divided into groups A and B, depending upon their capacity to be grown in cell culture and the pathological changes they produced in newborn mice.

The third group of ECHO viruses, which were also found to cause human type disease, were discovered and named as orphan viruses because the researchers did not know what disease they caused – so they were viruses looking for a home!

After the classification of the ECHO viruses, new enteroviruses were found and were given enterovirus numbers from 68 to 72 – so, in total, there are at least 72 now known and new ones are occasionally being added.

The way in which you can sub-type each one of these 72 viruses depends upon differences that occur in the structure of the VP1, VP2, VP3 and VP4 proteins in the viral shell. The way in which these proteins are made and are arranged on the surface gives rise to specific antibody response from the infected person, and that long-term IgG class antibody will only neutralize that particular virus. There is very little cross-reaction between each of the 72 enteroviruses, so it is the specific neutralizing effect of antibody that allows the identification of each of the 72 enteroviruses.

All of these enteroviruses have worldwide distribution and are extremely common. They cause widespread disease processes but have a specific propensity to attack muscle and brain tissue. They give rise, therefore, to a variation of the inflammatory disease of muscle called myositis or encephalitis (inflammation of the brain) and meningitis (inflammation of the lining of the brain). They can also cause paralysis and infections of the heart muscle (myocarditis), the pancreas (pancreatitis), the liver (hepatitis) and many other diseases. Usually, however, the disease process that they produce is a harmless one, a slight cold or a minor gastro-intestinal upset, because the common place of entry of the enteroviruses to the human body is through the mouth into the gut. Reproduction of the virus occurs in cells lining the gut, and also in the back of the throat, in the pharynx.

The majority of the enteroviruses, once the initial site of virus reproduction has evolved, pass into the bloodstream, and then involve their particular target organ, e.g. the brain, muscle, liver etc.

The incubation period between the initial infection and the development of the specific disease can vary from anything to two to forty days. Initially, the site of infection is probably in

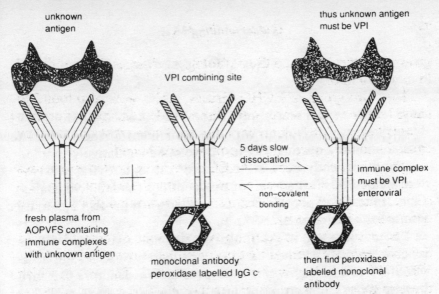

unknown antigen

thus unknown antigen must be VPI

VPI combining site

5 days slow dissociation

non–covalent bonding

immune complex must be VPI enteroviral

fresh plasma from AOPVFS containing immune complexes with unknown antigen

monoclonal antibody peroxidase labelled IgG c

then find peroxidase labelled monoclonal antibody

Fig. 4   Serological demonstration of enteroviral antigen
in immune complexes

the lymph nodes either in the gut or the throat, and also in the related lymphatic tissue in the tonsils or in the intestine itself. It is at this point that the virus can be found in large amounts either in the sputum from the mouth or in the faeces.

After this incubation period the virus is recoverable from the brain fluid, from the cerebro-spinal fluid if one develops an encephalitis, from nervous tissue or from muscle. The virus is capable of going to those specific areas because of the cell receptocytes, which match the protein structure of VP1, VP2, VP3 and VP4.

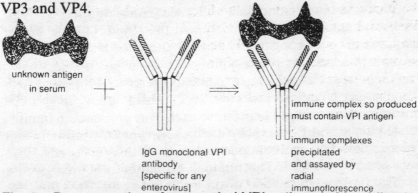

unknown antigen in serum

IgG monoclonal VPI antibody [specific for any enterovirus]

immune complex so produced must contain VPI antigen

immune complexes precipitated and assayed by radial immunoflorescence

Fig. 5   Demonstration of enteroviral VPI antigen in blood (basis
of M.E. Association test)

The VPI Test

M.E. sufferers can now apply to the M.E. Association for a VPI blood test, which is done with the agreement of their GP. The explanation of how this VPI test developed is relatively simple.

As has already been stated, all of the enteroviruses have a capsule and this is made up of polypeptides (amino acid chains). One of these polypeptide chains is called virus protein 1, and it is common to each one of the 72 enteroviruses, whereas other parts of the capsule are not. At St Mary's Hospital a very pure culture of Coxsackie B5 was heated to approximately 56°C for about ten minutes, and in this way it was possible to denature the virus protein capsule and strip out virus protein 1.

This particular polypeptide has a molecular weight of approximately 30,000 and is thus quite large. It is said to be antigenic – in other words, if virus protein 1 is put inside a human being, it will stimulate the immune system to make an antibody. However, there is something else that can be done with it – it can be used to make a monoclonal antibody specific to that virus protein 1. This antibody is extremely pure, and can be made in the laboratory along the following lines.

The technician takes the antigen of virus protein 1 and inoculates a laboratory mouse. This mouse's B-lymphocytes start making an antibody to that VPI. A sample of the lymphocytes is then separated so as to develop a single 'clone' – a specific line of cells.

This separated 'clone' line will make antibody specifically to VPI. The amount that it makes, and the length of time that it makes it in, is of course very limited, because after a few days or perhaps a week or so this white cell will die.

The white cell lymphocyte 'clone' is therefore hybridized with a malignant lymphoid cancerous cell, which of course has the unfortunate property of being immortal. This produces an immortalized malignant B-lymphocyte which, if cared for properly and fed appropriately, will continue to churn out this very specific and pure antibody to VPI. This monoclonal antibody is then given a peroxidase label (a flag) so it can be found again. Now the tests can be applied.

By taking a sample of the subject's blood and discarding the red cells, white cells and platelets – all of the solid particles within the blood – the technician is then left with a preparation of serum. A small portion of serum is then mixed with the anti-VPI monoclonal antibody. If there is any VPI in the blood, it will immediately stick to the anti-VPI monoclonal antibody and produce an immune complex. This complex can be precipitated and the amount produced can be estimated, so it is possible to measure the amount of precipitated VPI in the subject's blood.

We clearly had to be able to interpret what this meant, and we had to do control studies to be certain that this did not occur in healthy people, nor in other disease processes. First, there is a very, very small amount of VPI to be found in pooled serum from, say, 10,000 people. In order to establish a significant positive test in our subjects, we had to take several standard deviations above that level.

We also made comparisons with other diseases, and there did not appear to be another in which a persistent enterovirus VPI effect could be found. However, we know that it can occur as a positive result in healthy people, and it will be positive in a person who is in the first two or three days of an acute enterovirus infection, but not to any degree after that period of time. There also appears to be a higher level of VPI positive tests in children under the age of twelve, so it cannot be considered a reliable indicator here.

So what does a positive VPI test via the M.E. Association mean? It must not be taken to be a test for M.E.; it is not. What it does indicate is that at the time the positive blood sample was taken that person was actively suffering from an enterovirus infection. Where positive, it is an indicator that the diagnosis of M.E. should be considered, but it should be taken from a clinical point of view. If one could repeat the test on several occasions over a long period of time and it remained positive, that would mean that there was a persistent enterovirus infection; but unfortunately, we do not at the moment have the capability of offering more than just one test, so this test must be taken in context with the patient's clinical condition at the time.

As a result of positive VPI tests I have received many requests from GPs to see patients who are suffering from chronic symptoms which, from a clinical point of view, I find very difficult to assess. Patients are unfortunately using this as a positive test for M.E. and thus, correctly or incorrectly, believe they have the disease; equally, many patients are very disappointed when the test is negative, but I must point out that a negative test certainly does not exclude the diagnosis of either AOPVFS or M.E.

I have also noticed that the level of VPI in the blood of any one individual varies quite markedly from time to time. It seems to follow the clinical state of the patient – in other words, if the patient is very ill and actively getting worse, he or she has more virus protein 1 in the blood than if he or she is getting better or is not too unwell. So it is clearly important when the blood sample is taken because the test may, in the same patient, be positive one day and negative another. This is simply due to the fact that the antigen level fluctuates.

I have been taking four blood samples at fortnightly and three-weekly sampling times, and considering two positive results to indicate a persistent enterovirus infection. Unfortunately, logistics would make it extremely difficult, if not impossible, to offer four tests over a period of eight or twelve weeks to everybody suspected of having M.E.

The virological tests

As the vast majority of all virus infections – probably over 99 per cent of the type that we are talking about – get better within the first few days or certainly a week or so, specific virological tests are not often applied. This is especially so as there are no specific remedies for the majority of virus infections. So, fulfilling the law of supply and demand, because there is little demand for virological testing, there have been few tests developed.

This is now rapidly changing, and virological testing is improving as virus problems become more prevalent. When looking at the enteroviruses, the clinical picture tends to be that of a non-specific flu-like illness. There are dozens of viruses which will give the same clinical phenomena, and identifying exactly which one is involved can be very difficult; the techniques are often awkward and expensive, and are only infrequently available in a few centres dotted around the country. They are thus rarely done, except as an academic exercise, although enterovirus epidemics are studied at a research laboratory in Colindale, and other viruses which cause flu or cold-like symptoms are studied elsewhere in the south of England.

To be certain about which virus is involved in any type of infection, it is essential to recover active and infective virus. To do this it is usually necessary to take swabs from the nose, the throat, or the faeces within the first week or, at most, within ten days, and as complications in enterovirus infections are uncommon it is not at all likely that your doctor would be justified in doing such a test so early in the infection.

If AOPVFS is being considered, or complications arise from the initial infection, this is likely to happen after ten days, and it is probably no use taking swabs as by that stage the virus may well have gone, or be so heavily coated in antibody that its recovery from culture is unlikely. Consequently, when one is looking at problems associated with viruses two or three weeks after the initial infection, one is forced to look for other evidence of a virus effect.

As has already been explained, when a virus enters the body the immune system makes a specific antibody to that virus. The virus is neutralized and the body continues to demonstrate that antibody response; this response can be detectable. The immunological approaches discussed in more detail elsewhere depend upon the demonstration of long- and or short-term antibodies, which are referred to respectively as IgG and IgM.

An IgM response starts to occur in the blood after about a week or ten days. At this time detectable levels appear, and a normal person recovering from an enterovirus infection will demonstrate an IgM response for between three to twelve weeks, or even longer. The peak response is at about four to six weeks. This antibody response is detectable by a technique known as an ELISA (enzyme linked immunosorbent assay). This has only been developed in the last few years and is a very complicated technique, currently available in probably less than half a dozen centres in Great Britain, although these numbers are increasing.

The standardization of this test from one centre to another tends to vary, and therefore the interpretation of the result can alter, but a positive test is generally accepted by virologists as being indicative of 'evidence of a recent enterovirus infection'. This IgM ELISA test is not specific for one enterovirus – it cannot tell you whether your infection is due to Coxsackie B1, ECHO 19 or Coxsackie A12. It is a generalized response to all of them, and there is a large cross-reaction. This response is said to be heterotypic.

The test is not an all or nothing one – an IgM level at the beginning of an infection is very low in absolute terms. It then builds up to higher levels, before falling away. When it reaches a certain level it is considered to be positive. This level is predetermined by the laboratory involved, and is usually taken at either two or two and a half standard deviations above normal. It is said to have a 99 per cent confidence rating, and is at this level highly significant. However, in order to interpret what this means, one must of course compare it with levels found in the normal population, and here there appears to be a very variable interpretation.

Some studies done in Scotland suggest that there is a very high positive ELISA to the enteroviruses found in the normal population, whereas other studies done in the south of England show very much lower levels, and therefore a positive test here seems to have a greater clinical interpretation. What value we can place on a positive enterovirus IgM antibody response is still questionable and the result must not be taken out of context with the clinical picture.

IgG antiviral antibodies are long-term. They generally start to occur in the recovery phase, initially within two or three weeks, and they are very hard, which means they stay in the bloodstream at quite high detectable levels for many years. When found in a healthy person, they simply indicate an infection by a specific enterovirus at some stage in the past. Unlike the IgM response, the IgG response is specific for the virus involved – indeed, it is used in identifying each of the 72-odd types of enterovirus. An IgG response will be exact for, say, Coxsackie B3 or ECHO 19, and one can have a high level of confidence that the subject has been infected by those viruses in the past.

The problem lies in that latter statement – the IgG indicates a virus infection in the past, but it does not tell you what is happening now. Because the antibody response can last for many years we believe that these tests are quite uninterpretable, even if the IgG response is at a very high level.

The relationship between M.E. and its various forms has

Culture technique	AOPVFS patients (n=76)	Controls (n=30)
No of patients:		
After direct culture	2 (3%)	2 (7%)
Only after acid centrifugation	15 (20%)	0⋆
Total	17 (22%)	2 (6.7%)

*⋆AOPVFS vs controls: x^2=45.9, p<0.01.

Fig. 6   Virus isolation from faeces of AOPVFS patients
and controls

always been anecdotally related to the enterovirus group, and specifically Coxsackie B1–5. In years gone by it was the presence of high neutralizing IgG antibodies that formed the basis of this hypothesis but, while it is interesting to note that AOPVFS and M.E. have higher than usual IgG antibody responses, they are now considered of no help in the diagnosis of these conditions for the reasons given above.

Some virologists suggest that if you can show a sudden rise in this IgG response that would indicate a recent exposure to that virus; again, this is considered unreliable, as other immunological influences can alter the levels of these enterovirus IgG antibodies in the blood.

So these are the difficulties; viruses can only be easily grown in the first week or so of an infection; an IgM response, while indicating recent infection, can occur in quite large amounts in the normal population and the interpretation can be difficult; and levels of IgG long-term antibody are generally believed to be uninterpretable.

So how can we test for the presence of active enterovirus, which we believe is associated with M.E. and AOPVFS? The answer is really to be found in a persistently positive VPI test.

| | May 1986 | | | May 1987 | | |
Group	Isolate Direct	Isolate Acid centrifugation	VPI antigen	Acid centrifugation isolate	VPI antigen	Enterovirus-specific IgM antibody
PVFS:						
1	None	CB5	+	None	+	Heterotypic
2	None	Echo-1	+	None	-	-
3	None	CB2	+	CB2	+	Monotypic
4	CB5	CB5	-	None	-	-
5	None	CB3	+	None	+	Heterotypic
6	None	Echo-11	+	None	+	Heterotypic
7	None	CB1	+	CB1	+	Heterotypic
8	None	CB2	+	CB2	+	Monotypic
9	None	CB2	+	None	-	Monotypic
10	None	CB5	+	None	+	Heterotypic
11	None	CB4	+	None	-	Heterotypic
12	None	Echo-9	+	None	+	-
13	None	CB1	+	None	-	Heterotypic
14	None	Untyped	+	Untyped	+	Heterotypic
15	None	Untyped	+	None	-	Monotypic
16	Echo-11	Echo-11	-	None	+	-
17	None	CB4	+	CB4	+	Heterotypic
Controls:						
1	CB5	CB5	-	NT	-	NT
2	CB5	CB5	-	NT	-	NT

NT = not tested.

Fig.7 Correlation of results in 76 AOPVFS patients (Group A) and 30 controls in May 1986, and 12 months later

Do other viruses cause M.E. or AOPVFS?

My own view of M.E. is that it is a disease process in which a persistent enterovirus is the cause, so by definition M.E. is only caused by the enteroviruses. However, in AOPVFS patients I have been able to identify not only the enteroviruses, but also EBV. I have not at any stage been able to associate it virologically with any other virus. Anecdotally, however, I have four cases in which the patients told me that a classical herpes zoster initiated their problem – in other words, they had had shingles, and apparently nothing else.

I have discussed this with other physicians and have heard Dr Behan state that he has seen this phenomenon come on after chicken pox and several cases of rubella (German measles). However, no virological evidence has been put forward to substantiate those statements. I can appreciate that patients may develop a disease process subsequent to chicken pox as my patients did after shingles; those two viruses are herpes viruses, and they are capable of incorporation within the genetic material of the host gene, and of re-activation – shingles is in fact the reactivated virus of chicken pox. However, as far as I am aware rubella does not have a reactivated state.

My feeling is that AOPVFS is a disease process that is initiated by a virus; that disease process is immunologically determined and what we are detecting subsequently is a result of that disorder, not necessarily the cause of it. That statement allows that viruses other than the enteroviruses and EBV could precipitate the phenomenon.

To the question, 'Does anything else cause acute onset post viral fatigue syndrome?' the answer is emphatically 'No'. While we may not have a virological answer for some 30–35 per cent of AOPVFS, I certainly do not see that gap being filled by obscure suggestions such as an M.E. virus, spirochaetes, candida or the like.

The virological and immunological results found in patients with AOPVFS and M.E.

This study formed the basis of the paper published in the *Lancet* of 23 January 1988. Working on patients with AOPVFS, I submitted

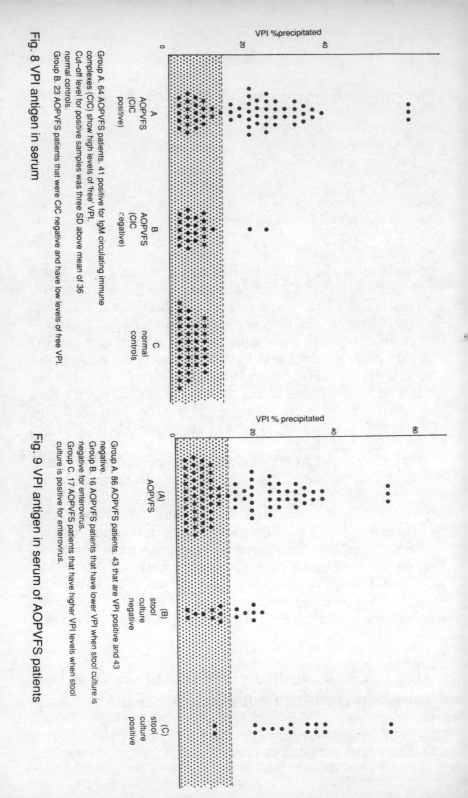

Fig. 8 VPI antigen in serum

Group A. 64 AOPVFS patients. 41 positive for IgM circulating immune complexes (CIC) show high levels of 'free' VPI.
Cut-off level for positive samples was three SD above mean of 36 normal controls.
Group B. 23 AOPVFS patients that were CIC negative and have low levels of free VPI.

Fig. 9 VPI antigen in serum of AOPVFS patients

Group A. 86 AOPVFS patients. 43 that are VPI positive and 43 negative.
Group B. 16 AOPVFS patients that have lower VPI when stool culture is negative for enterovirus.
Group C. 17 AOPVFS patients that have higher VPI levels when stool culture is positive for enterovirus.

blood and stool samples with age/sex match and geographically located controls to St Mary's Hospital for further analysis by the method of acid centrifugation. This showed that a large proportion of the group had evidence of a persistent enterovirus infection.

As will be seen from Fig.6, 22 per cent of the patients were found to have recoverable virus from their stool compared with 6.7 per cent of the control group. From a statistical point of view this has a very high significance (P being greater than 0.01).

The next step was find out what virus was present and so the viral deposits left after centrifugation were sent to Dr Eleanor Bell in Glasgow for culture and for identification. It can be seen from Fig.7 that eleven of these were a Coxsackie B virus, the others either being untyped or ECHO viruses.

In order to see whether this was just a one-off effect or not, we decided to repeat the whole process, using the same patients and the same controls, a year later, and the results are in the right-hand column of Fig.7. This time five of the patients grew virus – the same virus as was isolated the year before.

As is also shown in Fig.7, we looked for VPI antigen in the blood. On the left-hand side of the table can be seen a high correlation between VPI antigen and virus being present in the stool. The right-hand side shows that where virus was found a year later VPI antigen was also detected.

The Coxsackie B IgM by ELISA was also applied and, again on the right-hand side of the table, you will find a high correlation between virus VPI antigen present in the blood and a positive IgM antibody response.

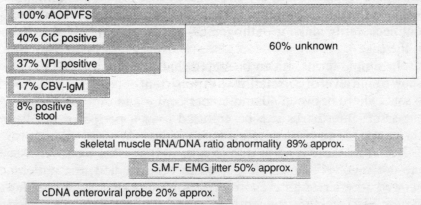

Fig. 10   Percentage relationship of enteroviral 'findings' seen in AOPVFS

IgM circulating immune complexes and enterovirus VPI in the serum

Looking at Fig.8, the vertical axis indicates the amount of VPI antigen that was found in the serum and the horizontal axis shows three separate groups studied, Groups A, B and C. Those in Group A had a diagnosis of AOPVFS and were IgM complex positive. It can be seen that in this group there were also high levels of precipitated VPI. Group B also had a diagnosis of AOPVFS but were found to be IgM complex negative with low levels of VPI in the serum. Group C were a control group of age/sex matched healthy people. The point to be noted here is that about two-thirds of AOPVFS patients studied (Group A) had high levels of enterovirus antigen VPI and were making short-term IgM immune complexes.

Fig.9 shows again on the vertical axis the amount of enterovirus VPI antigen in the blood and, on the horizontal axis, the comparison between the whole group of AOPVFS (Group A), and those in which there was an enterovirus that was grown or not (Groups B and C) after by acid centrifugation. Here one can see that there was a higher detectable amount of VPI in the blood in those who had a recoverable enterovirus from the faeces.

So what did all of this mean? It all leads to sound scientific evidence that patients who are suffering from AOPVFS have evidence for a persistent enterovirus in their body. At present we are not able to state that the virus is the cause of that phenomenon – the fact that we can detect it in the faeces and in the blood does not necessarily make it pathogenic – but it seems likely that that is the case.

In simple terms, it can be stated that patients with AOPVFS show a high level of correlation with persistent enterovirus infection – somewhere between 40 and 60 per cent – and on faecal testing the same enterovirus can be cultured over a period of not less than a year. The viruses isolated are not just Coxsackie B but also ECHO, and there is no reason to suggest that other enteroviruses are not involved. Over the period of time studied, the patients showed free circulating enterovirus antibody that their immune system was making; the antigen and the antibody were joined

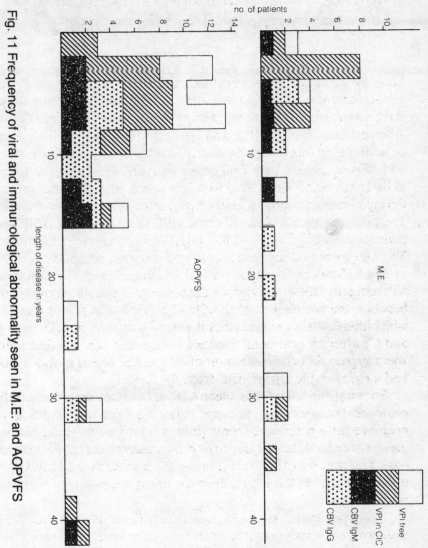

Fig. 11 Frequency of viral and immunological abnormality seen in M.E. and AOPVFS

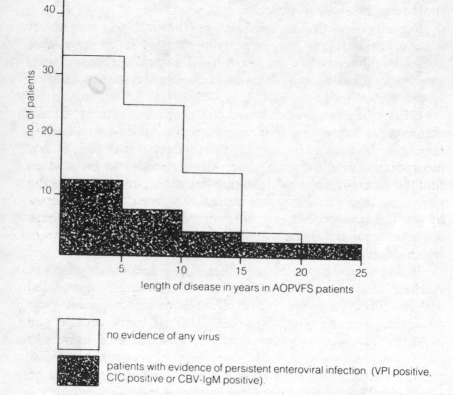

length of disease in years in AOPVFS patients

no evidence of any virus

patients with evidence of persistent enteroviral infection. (VPI positive, CIC positive or CBV-IgM positive).

Recovery in both groups appears to be similar. About half the patients have recovered in ten years.

Fig .12   Demonstration that clinical improvement
occurs irrespective
of presence of virus

together in the immune complexes, and those immune complexes contained enterovirus.

The story of what is happening might, then, go something like this.

At the beginning of the disease process, the patient develops an enterovirus infection; the virus multiplies in the gut, and becomes persistent there. The gut supplies a constant source of reinfection, and that reinfection is seen by the detection of virus particles in the blood, and the fact that the body is continuously making a short-term antibody to that virus.

We also know that enterovirus can be found in muscle and it is not unreasonable to suggest that those same viral elements that are found in the muscle also occur in the central nervous system, accounting for the preponderance of muscle and central nervous system symptoms found in M.E. and AOPVFS.

Unlike the Epstein Barr virus, which can reactivate or become chronic, the enteroviruses have no known mechanism whereby they can become latent, and their genetic material is not incorporated into the host gene. Consequently, to be able to find the enteroviruses, the infection has to be persistent, and the virus must be constantly reproducing. Until recently the processes by which this may occur have not been understood, but now there are several animal models and in-vitro cultures and cell lines in which this can be achieved.

It can be seen from Fig.10 that if one takes any group of AOPVFS patients a proportion of them are clearly associated with evidence for persistent enterovirus. Forty per cent show circulating immune complexes (CIC) that are based on IgM and in which the antigen can frequently be demonstrated to be VPI enterovirus in origin. A large proportion of those that are CIC positive also have evidence of free circulating VPI antigen, which is not complexed, and a further proportion of those are enterovirus IgM free circulating antibody positive, which is also not complexed as assayed by ELISA. A further subset of the latter group are enterovirus positive for faecal culture.

Last, but by no means least, we know that there is a group in which enterovirus RNA can be seen within the cells of skeletal muscle, but as yet I am not sure exactly in what number that abnormality is found.

This still leaves quite a large proportion of AOPVFS patients in which there is no direct relationship with persistent enterovirus. At the time of doing this study there was certainly no evidence to suggest any other causative viral agent; the EBV relationship did not occur until much later.

In the upper graph of slow onset M.E. (see Fig.11) some thirty patients were studied and 74 per cent were found to have CICs containing IgM in which the antigen was found to be enterovirus related. Their free circulating VP1 was not assessed in this study. Twenty-two per cent of them were found to have high neutralizing antibody to Coxsackie B virus of greater than 1:256, compared with less than 3 per cent of age/sex/match controls. However, while this appeared to be significant it was not statistically so.

Enterovirus IgM by ELISA was found to be statistically significant and its interpretation is one of evidence of recent or persistent infection.

The lower graph in Fig.11 measuring the same markers shows the distribution as found in the AOPVFS and from a statistical point of view there seems to be very little difference in the virological and immunological responses between the two groups. This is a very significant finding, as it suggests that the same virological processes are going on in M.E. and AOPVFS, although there appears to be more evidence of an enterovirus relationship in the slow onset type than there is in the acute phenomenon.

Looking at the two graphs, there does not appear to be a tendency for free circulating IgM to be found at the beginning of the disease, but it is found during it. This suggests that these antibodies are not resulting from recent infection, but are more likely to be due to a persistent production of antibody (see Fig.12).

When one looks at the symptomatology of AOPVFS and slow onset M.E. there appears to be very little to distinguish between the two, except possibly at the very beginning of the disorder, when some of the malaise and psychiatric symptoms are more prevalent in AOPVFS. The virological and immunological results also show very little difference between the two. This leads to the interesting concept that the two disease processes are actually the same.

In the chapter on immunology I explained that there are different types of white cell to be found in the bloodstream, some of which are lymphocytes divided into two groups – T cells and B cells. The T cells are further divided into sub groups called, for example, T4 and T8. There is a known ratio of these T cells and a particular shift in this ratio would indicate possibly an acute virus infection or a chronic one.

Dr Behan's research suggests that there were significant abnormalities in these ratios, specifically in T4/8 ratios. However, after looking at some forty-five AOPVFS patients and also a number of slow onset M.E. in my patient group I came to the conclusion that there were no abnormalities in the sub group studied.

The results of a generalized virological screen were the next thing to consider. Serum samples from all of those studied, including the control group, were tested for various types of antibody responses to some of our common viruses, including herpes simplex (cold sores), herpes zoster (shingles) varicella (chicken pox), measles, mumps, the adeno viruses, the respiratory syncytial virus, the influenza viruses A and B and the para influenza viruses.

The results were quite remarkable, in that there was not one suggestion of even a slightly abnormal antibody response that could implicate any virus mentioned in the list above. We did consider the Epstein Barr virus and we assumed that a negative EBV serology looking for the short-term antibody IgM would rule out that possibility. We did not then appreciate that other antibody responses should be considered, which became apparent in later study of the disease complex.

During our biochemical assessment, we also looked at CPK (creatine phospho-kinase). This is an enzyme which occurs in skeletal muscle and, if there is any damage to that muscle, it tends to leak into the bloodstream and is detectable by a rise in CPK. We found that there was no rise in CPK in either AOPVFS or in slow onset M.E. This would indicate that there is no evidence of any destructive or significant tissue damage.

Early in the study I sent samples of blood to the Middlesex Hospital, where Dr Jonathan Brostoff was kind enough to look for free circulating IgE and IgE complexes. This immunoglobulin class is often found to be abnormal in people who are suffering from various types of allergic phenomena. All of the serum submitted was normal, and there was no suggestion of any true allergic response except in one patient with a history of hay fever; her blood was taken in May and June when her symptoms were particularly severe and there was a significant rise in her free circulating IgE.

We were not able to study any particular immunological abnormalities with regard to candida albicans. There are tests that are available to show IgE and IgM responses to this yeast, and this is something that I will be looking at in the near future with Dr Brostoff, who has been kind enough to offer this facility.

7

THE EPSTEIN BARR VIRUS

This ubiquitous virus is perhaps the commonest of all to infect man, and once present it is there for life. It is contracted by droplet spread – an infected person coughs or breathes the virus out in small droplets of sputum which drift across the atmosphere to an uninfected person. The inoculation of infected mucus within the nose, throat and mucous membranes is the usual site of entry.

EBV is known to be associated with, and probably the causative agent of, several different diseases, including two well recognized malignancies – Burkitts lymphoma and nasopharyngeal carcinoma. It is well established to be reactivated in some serious immune compromised situations such as AIDS or organ transplantation.

Its commonest infection is probably quite asymptomatic in the very young, but it later causes infectious mononucleosis or glandular fever and, because it stays in the nucleus of the cells forever, it can be reactivated in situations of immune compromisation.

In 1964 there was worldwide interest in Burkitts lymphoma, which is one of the commonest childhood cancers found in Africa. The story had started in the 1950s when Mr Dennis Burkitt, a British surgeon working in Uganda, came across a young lad who had a rather strange malignant tumour, which proved to be a white cell tumour, called a lymphoma. This tumour proved to be devastatingly fast in growth capability, being able to double its size in thirty-six hours, and was rapidly fatal. After a lot of detective work, Burkitt found that this particular tumour had a seasonal variation, and a geographical phenomenon that suggested there could be a relationship between it and mosquito transmission of malaria.

In later years, some biopsies of Burkitts lymphoma were looked at under an electron microscope at the Middlesex Hospital in London by Messrs Epstein, Achong and Barr. They found inside the cells viral particles which, after cooperation with Drs Henle and Henle in America, were found to be a new herpes virus. In 1966 Henle and Henle discovered that people developed antibodies to this virus while suffering from infectious mononucleosis (IM) and later EBV was shown to be the sole viral agent implicated in IM, although it was not present in all cases. In the same year Dr Old *et al.* found that EBV was a direct co-factor in the genesis of a nasty cancer of the nose and pharynx common in southern China.

Like the enteroviruses, the herpes viruses are structurally extremely similar to one another, but the herpes viridae as a family is vast, and new ones are continually being found. They are all double standard deoxyribonucleic acid (DNA) encapsulated viruses, they are all icosahedral (twenty-sided) and they are quite large at over 100 nanometres in diameter. The capsid is made up of 162 hollow capsomeres.

An envelope, or membrane, lies around the outside of the capsid and is derived from the cell that it infects, and makes up the total diameter of the virus as being in excess of 150–200 nm. There are four major herpes viruses which cause disease: Herpes simplex virus (HSV), of which there are two types, HSV1 and HSV2. These cause herpes; herpes varicella – zoster virus (VZV) which causes chicken pox and shingles; cytomegalo virus (CMV), which causes congenital defects and diseases in immuno-suppressed patients; and Epstein Barr virus (EBV). Human herpes virus 6 (HHV6), which has only just been discovered, is not, as yet, associated with a disease.

The Epstein Barr virus is the same shape as the other herpes viruses, and looks just like the diagram in fig 13. It is a large virus, being probably three to four times bigger in capsular size than the enteroviruses, and up to ten times bigger if you include the lipid

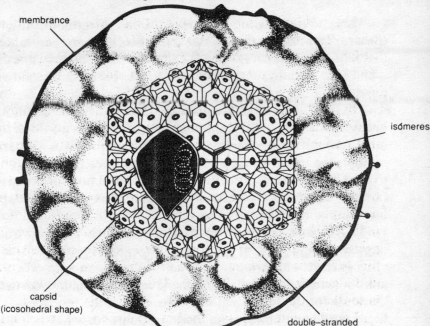

membrane

isómeres

capsid
(icosohedral shape)

double–stranded
DNA genome

Fig. 13   The Epstein Barr Virus

membrane. It has a molecular weight of 100×10^6 Daltons.

The DNA double strand has a molecular weight of about 180 kilo bases, that is, it has 180,000 nucleotide bases in various orders and sequences that have the virus genetic code capability and the whole sequence of the viral DNA molecule is now known. During infection the viral DNA is found to be inside the host cell nucleus, where it exists in two forms. Some of the viral DNA is integrated into the host cell chromosomes, into the cells' genetic material, and thus, whenever that cell divides, virus sequences can be found in daughter cells. It therefore has the capability of being redeveloped at any time. The majority of the virus DNA, however, is near, but not incorporated into, the chromosome and is found in little circular molecules.

One important feature of EBV is that it has a specific affinity for the receptors found on B-lymphocytes and so far, apart from epithelial cells, seems only able to infect these particular lymphocytes. It is not known whether the virus can penetrate any other cell – for instance, it cannot get inside a brain cell or skeletal muscle.

This affinity for white cells forms the basis of the ability to culture the virus in the laboratory. However, the technique is very laborious and requires the separation of B-cells from the blood obtained from a placenta – equivalent, therefore, to newborn baby blood which has never been exposed to EBV – and inoculating this product with EBV. The infected B-cells then undergo a transformation and become immortal, unlike uninfected B-cells which would normally die. In the test tube these virus-infected B-lymphocytes will carry on multiplying and can form a permanent cell line. These cells appear to lose their natural growth control in an almost pre-malignant fashion, and this may be one of the explanations for the virus being involved in malignant disease.

The various breaking up products of such a large virus are numerous, and most of them are antigenic – in other words, the virus particle will turn on the B-cells to make an antibody. These antibodies can be detected and the levels at which they occur form the basis for the individual laboratory tests; the interpretation of these various antibody responses accounts for what is going on inside the body in the various stages of EBV.

In the case of EBV, the initial antibody response that is produced by the B-cells is non-specific. The Epstein Barr virus stimulates the B-cells to make all kinds of antibody, and this non-specific antibody response is referred to as heterotypic. A blood test can be done to look for this non-specific heterophile antibody. There is a second portion of this non-specific antibody response that is associated with a positive Paul Bunnell test that occurs at this stage of the infection starting from about the tenth day. These blood tests have been thought to be specific; however, I have had patients who have given positive non-specific heterophile antibody and Paul Bunnell tests but, when I have looked for more exact antibody responses, such as a VCAIgG, have proved never to have been exposed to EBV. Consequently a more specific marker for the disease must be sought, and that is the atypical monocyte response.

Once a single Epstein Barr virus has penetrated a B-lymphocyte, it leaves a surface marker at the point of penetration. This is referred to as lymphocyte detected membrane antigen (LYDMA). The LYDMA possesses a remarkable property in that it causes a non-specific turn-on of T-cells, and this is termed an atypical monocytic response. These T-cells are very active, and mature into killer cells which start knocking out virus infective B-cells. Once this happens Epstein Barr virus antibodies start to appear in the blood.

One of the first antibody responses, called a viral capsid antigen response, is to the Epstein Barr virus capsule. At the beginning, this will be a short-term antibody response and therefore will be an IgM antibody. However, as recovery starts this viral capsid antigen response will turn into an IgG antibody – the long-term antibody response. As this IgG antibody strengthens, the patient recovers. The IgG antibody level then stabilizes and remains in that person for life.

In the early stages of the infection, one would also expect to find other antibody responses. The early antigen response (EA) is a particular antibody which is known to indicate an active virus cycle. A little later, in the recovery period, the hard nuclear antibodies start to appear; there are called Epstein Barr nuclear antigen antibodies (EBNA). Their precise role is not understood, but they also stabilize and their appearance indicates recovery.

Over the next few weeks, and probably even months, this primary infection begins to settle. The virus being shed from the mouth diminishes but continues to be produced from the epithelium of the pharynx for ever; even in healthy people EBV can be found to be shed in the saliva in varying levels.

Within the bloodstream one can find a trickle of virus going into the system, probably from the epithelium of the pharynx, which infects the occasional B-cell. This B-cell will then be challenged by a memory T-cell, which then matures into a killer cell and knocks out the infected B-cell. Thus, within the recovered state, there develops a status quo of virus infecting B-cells, B-cells being killed by T-cells.

The immunological response also balances itself out. A stable viral capsid antigen IgG response occurs, the early antigen disappears, usually to undetectable levels, and the nuclear antigens EBNA 1 and 2 stabilize at detectable levels. In the recovered individual, there will be no viral capsid antigen IgM response, which may in other situations suggest a continuing EBV infection.

The resulting delicately balanced immune response is remarkably stable, and within any one group of recovered persons the VCAIgG and the EBNA levels remain very constant. The whole picture can be observed and taken as a barometer of immune competence.

It is clear from studying normal control populations and healthy individuals that there is quite a large range to be found in these antibody values, suggesting different levels of immune surveillance. Some have a rather inefficient T-killer cell surveillance, and here higher levels of VCAIgG and lower levels of EBNA 1 are found; in others that appear to have a much tighter control, very low levels of VCAIgG and higher levels of EBNA 1 are seen. Sometimes, in the less tight T-cell surveillance group, one might even find low levels of detectable early antigen.

When trying to establish the role of EBV in any subsequent disease process, actually isolating the virus, either in the blood or in the throat, is of no help because it is there all the time in normal people. It is looking at various antibodies and the levels of those antibodies that gives one insight into what might be happening. It is known that various EBV antibody levels may be disturbed by many other disease processes. One should also remember that when looking at healthy people there is a large range of values found in the antibody response VCAIgG and also of levels of EBNA and, when looking at evidence for alterations of these viral antibodies, one must be prepared to compare EBV antibody findings not only in post viral syndrome, but other acute virus infections and other chronic illnesses to see what happens there. There are many internationally accepted criteria to the interpretation of these antibody levels and responses, but there is still a lot to learn about this ubiquitous virus.

Epstein Barr viral nuclear antigen (EBNA)

These are found to occur in patients who have an Epstein Barr virus infection and in whom recovery has taken place. At least four EBNA have been detected, and there are probably more. EBNA 1 and EBNA 2 are the better understood of these.

Membrane Antigen (MA)

The overlying membrane surrounding the virus capsule is a complex of at least three antigens. The membrane is necessary for the herpes virus to be infective and without it, it is neutralized. The membrane antigen itself is acquired when the virus destroys the host cell and it is derived from some of the cytoplasmic parts of the cell and the cell membrane.

Early Antigen (EA)

This antigen is only found when a virus-infected cell is destroyed and broken open. Its presence is known to represent an active reproduction phase of the virus. High levels indicate a high level of viral replication which is called a viral lytic cycle, lytic meaning the breaking down of host cell membrane.

EB viral capsid antigen (VCA)

This antigen is always found to be present in patients who have been exposed to a past infection. A viral capsid antigen old antibody response would be an IgG response, an active infection would be seen to contain a viral capsid antigen IgM response.

Lymphocyte detected membrane antigen (LYDMA)

This antigen is present on the surfaces of virus-infected cells. It allows specific T-cells to identify an infected cell and to kill it appropriately.

Who has EBV?

Several studies have been carried out, looking for the presence of the antibody responses mentioned above in normal healthy people, and it is surprising to note that over 92 per cent of the British population has been exposed to the Epstein Barr virus. This is shown by measuring levels of viral capsid antigen IgG in the blood of normal individuals. When lecturing, I ask how many members of the audience have been told that they have had glandular fever, and usually about 10 per cent put up their hands. Consequently 80 per cent of an average audience has been exposed to EBV, but it has not caused them a recognizable illness.

Studies have shown that by the age of 10, just under 50 per cent of us have had an EBV infection. Presumably this has either been quite subclinical, in other words not causing any symptoms at all, or has simply been just another minor cold or upper respiratory tract type of infection which would never have been recognized as EBV.

By the time that we have reached the age of twenty, 92 per cent of us have had a specific infection, and it is within this group, between the ages of twelve and twenty, that most of us experience that disease called infectious mononucleosis or glandular fever.

The reason why we get glandular fever as a specific disease process in our teens and yet do not get any recognizable illness in the younger years is not at all clear.

The picture of EBV infection in the western world is different from that of less well sanitized countries and poorer nations, where the 90 per cent infection total is achieved much earlier, presumably due to poor hygiene and overcrowded conditions.

Glandular fever

Although probably 90 per cent of glandular fever is caused by Epstein Barr virus, other viruses have been implicated. It starts with malaise, ill-health, pyrexia, widespread aches and pains and general flu-like symptoms, but a very severe sore throat occurs in the majority of people, along with glandular enlargement and tenderness, initially in the neck, but also under the armpits and in the groin. There is often enlargement of the liver and the spleen, because of the B-cells concentrated there; an enlarged spleen occurs in about 50 per cent of cases, while slightly more get an enlarged liver. Because of the involvement of the liver, a jaundice can occur. Skin rashes are not uncommon.

Sometimes the disease can progress even further and involve the brain, the heart or the lungs in an inflammatory process, and thus glandular fever is far from a mild illness. As already mentioned, it typically affects the teenager, and is probably caused here by the transmission of saliva by kissing. Hence it has often been referred to as the kissing disease.

In the normal course of events, several weeks are required for recovery, but it is not unusual to find people still feeling unwell after nine months or even a year.

The Epstein Barr virus group

Only 40 per cent of AOPVFS is accounted for by tests that demonstrate a persistent enterovirus infection and, while negative blood tests do not prove that one is not there, no matter how often I tested the blood the other 60 per cent of patients never demonstrated an enterovirus effect. Equally, when applying other routine viral screens, I could not detect any other virus.

The story of an acute onset and probably a virus type of start was clear, and was always exactly the same. My patients had the same symptoms, the same clinical progress and the same clinical picture, so arguably the disease process was the same. What was the explanation in the other 60 per cent?

A group of about 15 per cent of my AOPVFS patients were told by their GPs at the beginning of their disease that they were suffering from classical glandular fever. Tests had sometimes confirmed this but other patients having the typical clinical picture gave blood tests that had not supported this diagnosis. After their 'glandular fever' had gone on for several months, further tests did not show any evidence for the persistence of glandular fever, and the blood picture apparently returned to normal. Yet the patient had continued to feel ill, with symptoms suggestive of AOPVFS. So was this a chronic glandular fever type illness?

I consulted Dr Dorothy Crawford, Senior Lecturer in Virology at the Hammersmith Hospital, who is accepted by all virologists as being an expert in EBV. At our first interview, she expressed surprise that I did not think that AOPVFS was associated with EBV, as she had been testing the blood of many other people in this clinical group and was convinced there was a connection. She told me that she was just embarking upon a study of exactly that type, and that if I sent her a series of bloods from my patients she would analyse them and let me know what there was to find.

Just before the end of September 1987, I sent her 120 samples of blood from a group of patients of whom the clinical status was well established, and consisted of either M.E. or AOPVFS. This group consisted of approximately 40 per cent enteroviral association and

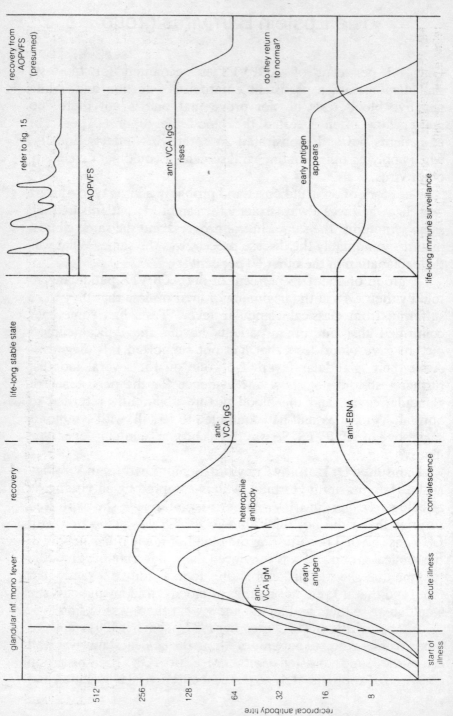

Fig. 14 Epstein Barr virus antiviral antibody levels in relationship to time after onset of 'glandular fever'

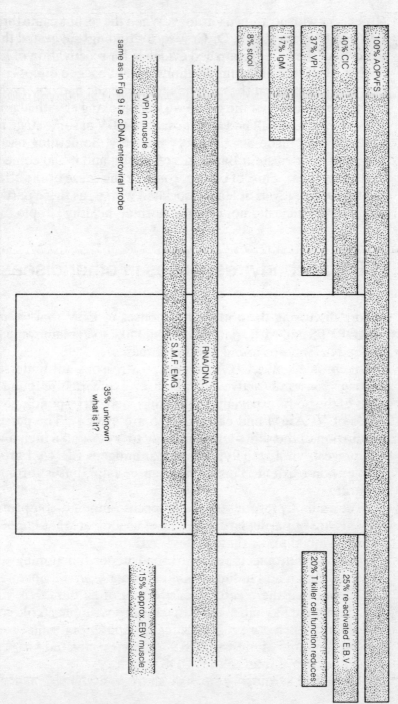

Fig. 15 Percentage of various abnormalities in AOPVFS and their relative position within that syndrome

100% AOPVFS

40% CIC

37% VPI

17% IgM

8% stool

same as in Fig 9 i.e. cDNA enteroviral probe

VPI in muscle

RNA/DNA

S.M.F. EMG

35% unknown
what is it?

25% re-activated E.B.V.

20% T killer cell function reduces

15% approx. EBV muscle

60 per cent with no known virology. When the results came through I was quite taken aback; Dr Crawford's findings suggested that 25 per cent of the latter group had evidence for reactivation of EBV.

Not at all sure of the implications, I went back to discuss it with her. She told me that the antibody response she had observed had led her to believe that the group we were looking at with abnormal EBV serology had all had an exposure to EBV at some stage in the past, and had made a satisfactory recovery. Something had now triggered their Epstein Barr virus off again, and it had come back to reinfect them. This, of course, could be the cause or the effect of their disorder; it was at least associated with it, as these particular antibody findings did not occur in normal, healthy people.

EBV antibody responses in other diseases

Before discussing the antibody responses to EBV that we found in AOPVFS and M.E. patients I would like to explain some EBV antibody responses found in other diseases.

In chronic active EBV the virus, for reasons not understood, becomes constantly active. Very high levels of virus are found in all parts of the body, especially in the lungs, and correspondingly high levels of VCAIgM and early antigen are evident. The persistent production of the short-term antibody to VCA and a high level of EA suggests viral activity; the nuclear antigens EBNA 1 are very low, or non-existent. This disease can be fatal, but is fortunately very rare.

The antibody responses seen in specific immuno-compromised patients are of particular interest. Let us look at what happens in the most infamous of these states – AIDS.

In this syndrome there is a broad under-functioning of the immune system and a diminution in immune surveillance. There is evidence that there can be reactivation of all the DNA viruses that the patient has had in the past and herpes simplex (cold sores), varicella (chicken pox) zoster (shingles) and cytomegalic virus are frequently found along with EBV. These reactivated viruses can sometimes prove fatal to the AIDS patient.

The EBV serology here will show a VCAIgG, a negative

VCAIgM, a rise in early antigen response and diminished EBNA 1. If VCAIgM response is negative that indicates there is not an active persistent infection, and that the problem in the AIDS patient did not start with a primary EBV infection, but a secondary reactivation. The antibodies to the other viruses show similar reactivation patterns.

The same phenomenon is noticed in other immuno-compromisation conditions. In transplant patients, the whole immune system is suppressed by drugs such as Cyclosporin and steroids in order to reduce the chance of rejection of the new organ. Antibody responses to incorporated viruses such as EBV also show a negative VCAIgM, a raised VCAIgG, a raised EA, and diminished EBNA 1.

EBV antibody response and its interpretation in AOPVFS

The following antibody responses are internationally accepted as being evidence of reactivation of EBV: a negative short-term VCAIgM response, a normal or raised long-term VCAIgG response, and an early antigen EA response of greater than 32, with a statistical lowering of EBNA 1. This is exactly what we found in the 25 per cent of patients suffering from AOPVFS, but not in patients associated with persistant enterovirus infection.

This suggests that the patients suffered from an EBV infection at some stage in the past, either asymptomatically or in the form of glandular fever, but made a normal recovery. Now they have reactivated their EBV virus, which implies there is something in their immune system that is not as efficient as it used to be.

Can primary glandular fever (EBV) cause AOPVFS?

The answer to this lies in being able to identify the virus infection at the beginning of the disease process of AOPVFS. Most of my patients come one, two, three or even four years after their initial problem, and their virus was frequently not established at the start. There is no chance of detecting that virus years later except by interpreting antibody responses.

In order to find out whether EBV is associated with the initial disease, I wrote to all the people with evidence for reactivation of EBV as carried out by Dr Crawford's blood tests and asked them to discuss with their doctors whether any blood tests had been done at the beginning of their illness, specifically tests looking for glandular fever. Had they had a Paul Bunnell or a heterophile antibody that was positive? Did they have a film looking for atypical monocytes? I asked for photocopies of these blood tests and results. I also enquired whether they had ever had a well-documented glandular fever illness prior to the onset of AOPVFS.

I was very pleased with the response; well over 50 per cent of them had had tests done at the beginning of their AOPVFS. Some had shown a positive Paul Bunnell but a negative atypical monocytes response – in other words, they had had some of the criteria for diagnosing EBV but there seems to have been a doubt as to whether this was a true EBV infection or some other kind of peculiar Paul Bunnell response. Others showed incontrovertible evidence of EBV infection well before the onset of their current AOPVFS, in that they had had both a positive Paul Bunnell and atypical monocyte response documented years previously.

However, there were several who had a positive Paul Bunnell and atypical monocyte response at the very beginning of their AOPVFS. They had had an EBV infection and continued to suffer from their disease; they now had a viral capsid antigen IgG response, and their viral capsid IgM antibody had gone negative. It will take a lot more work before we can clearly differentiate between these various virological diseases, antibody responses and processes which clinically seem to be the same.

On learning about the reactivation of EBV in AOPVFS and AIDS, some patients may wonder if they have some kind of immune deficiency problem. This is possible, but let me point out immediately that AIDS is caused by a specific virus and the resulting disease is a severe progressive destruction of the total immune response whereby death appears inevitable. If there is an immune deficiency problem in the reactivated EBV AOPVFS then it is far more specific and, as we know from the clinical picture, usually improves.

In AIDS, there is evidence of reactivation of all the DNA viruses, herpes simplex, zoster, CMV etc., whereas the antibody response to those viruses in AOPVFS stays within normal limits. This suggests, therefore, that in AOPVFS there is a specific deficiency to the virus versus host balance of the Epstein Barr virus.

We need still to establish whether reactivation of EBV occurs in other chronic disease processes, such as other virus infections or multiple sclerosis, before we can really begin to understand the part EBV plays in the whole concept of M.E. and AOPVFS.

Specific T-Killer cell dysfunction in reactivated EBV

Studies that have been done in Japan and America suggest that there is a natural T-killer cell dysfunction in some forms of chronic active EBV and we have already started looking at this facet within AOPVFS.

There is some suggestion that in AOPVFS the mechanism whereby the T-killer cells seek out the occasional infected B cell and knock it out is not working properly, so I have taken three groups of people for study. One group has the clinical AOPVFS with suggestion of reactivation of EBV; another has the same clinical AOPVFS but with evidence of a persistent enterovirus infection; and a third group is of age/sex matched normal controls. I have taken some fresh samples of blood from the three groups and then, by a very careful mechanism of ultra centrifugation, we have separated out the various B-cells and T-cells. We have then put the B-cells into a culture medium and infected the remaining uninfected B-cells with Epstein Barr virus; the next step is to reintroduce the patient's T-cells from another sample of blood. If the T-cells recognize the infected B-cells, the T-memory cells will convert into T-killer cells and kill the infected B-cells.

This technique is known as a regression assay, and we are finding that in patients with AOPVFS it does appear to show a specific deficiency of the T-killer cell function. This is not absolute – the infected B-cells are still killed, but not as efficiently as in healthy people.

In reactivated EBV there is an increased production of virus in the pharynx, an increased out-put of EBV from the mouth in sputum, and a commensurate increased uptake of EBV into the bloodstream. There are probably additional numbers of infected B-cells circulating in the system, and these cells are not being adequately destroyed by the T-killer cells, which have a specific deficiency now against these infected cells. It is possible, therefore, that the increased number of infected B-cells that appear to have a longer circulating life can mature, freshly made virus can be spilled into the bloodstream and the patient now suffers from a chronic reactivated EBV infection.

Other explanations for the antibody responses to EBV in post viral syndrome

To help me understand the unusual EBV antibody responses a little further, I went to Birmingham to discuss my problems with Professor Alan Rickinson, an expert in EBV virology. He told me that he had found a large group of healthy people who had similar antibody responses to those that I had found in AOPVFS – not quite so consistently abnormal as in my group, but certainly abnormal. He suggested that it reflected a wide range of normal virus versus host balance – that in those individuals who had a very tight and efficient T-killer cell activity, the levels of viral capsid antigen IgG and early antigen would be low, and in those with less efficient, but still normal, T-cell monitoring systems, there might be an unusually high VCAIgG response, and a high early antigen.

One explanation he offered was that when post viral syndrome develops, the whole of the T-killer cell monitoring system may be shifted to a less vigilant activity, and allow the VCAIgG and early antigen responses to shift to higher levels. He accepted that there was something significant in the antibody responses that I had found, but he did not necessarily feel they represented reactivation – rather that there might be a weakening of the T-cell response as a whole, caused by immunological or other physiological deficiencies.

The suggestion was made that we should compare these abnormal findings of EBV serology in AOPVFS with the EBV serology that might be found in other chronic fatigue syndromes of known neurological cause, such as multiple sclerosis, and also in acute virus infections that were not initially EBV. In other words, we shall look at EBV antibody responses in true influenza and in the common cold to see if this shift to suggest reactivation of EBV is in fact a specific finding in AOPVFS and not in other diseases.

We also discussed the possibility of these abnormal EBV antibody responses being those of a true chronic EBV infection. Professor Rickinson had several cases of a true chronic glandular fever or infectious mononucleosis syndrome caused by Epstein Barr virus – tests right at the beginning of the disease confirmed this. He thought it quite likely that at least a proportion of the group I was looking at could be suffering from chronic EBV and that the absence of VCAIgM response now did not exclude the possibility of AOPVFS being initially caused by EBV.

One factor that seems to make it unlikely, however, that the causative virus is EBV is the very late age onset. Primary EBV occurs in some 90 per cent of people by the age of 21, and to get an initial EBV infection at thirty-two, the peak age for AOPVFS seems improbable, although possible. If possible, it may be that the sequellae of a primary EBV infection in the later years is that of the development of AOPVFS.

With the increasing evidence that there are specific T-killer cell dysfunction, and EBV serology suggesting a generalized shift in the virus versus host balance, the possibility that AOPVFS is caused by some immunological upset, rather than the actual virus, must also be considered.

Let us take another scenario. There is no doubt that the disease process we are looking at suggests a virus start – it may be EBV, it may be one of the 72 enteroviruses, it may be another virus. Let us say that with the initial infection some deregulatory mechanism occurs and allows the development of an immuno-compromised state. Because of that immuno-comprised state, reactivation of EBV occurs, or a persistent enterovirus infection develops, so that the disease is actually an immunological one, and not primarily caused by the virus that is now detected.

It is clearly important to establish the truth of this theory, because if the presence of a virus indicates that that virus is the cause of the disease, then the patient can be cured by eradicating it. If, on the other hand, the virus is simply there because of the disease, then killing the virus will not make the patient better. For the former case we would need to develop specific antiviral remedies to kill the virus, for the latter some immuno-regulatory 'kick' to restore what may be a damaged immune system.

It is going to take a lot of very careful work to unravel these possibilities before embarking upon possible treatment programmes.

The association of EBV related AOPVFS and enterovirus related AOPVFS

I was interested to see whether any of my 40 per cent of AOPVFS patients associated with persistent enterovirus infection and 25 per cent associated with reactivated EBV had both viruses present. From our study, it became quite clear that they were two virologically very distinct groups. However, there was this interesting abnormality of a natural killer cell dysfunction. Did it only apply to the EBV group?

Our initial findings are that some of the samples we looked at for killer cell activity in the enterovirus group appear to have the same deficiency as that seen in the reactivated EBV group. These are very preliminary observations and further investigation is required, because once again the possibility is raised that while the virus is not actually causing the disease, the very nature of the disease allows the persistence of an enterovirus or the reactivation of the Epstein Barr virus.

8
WHERE IS THE DISEASE AND WHAT IS GOING ON?

Introduction

In order to develop a sensible treatment and management programme and to help direct future research one's initial work should be to try to understand precisely what is going on in any particular disease process. In M.E. and AOPVFS the majority of treatment programmes are purely anecdotal and unproven. The majority are not even sensible, and until we know what is happening I suppose there is no real reason why they should work. There are currently 5,000 cures for M.E!

There is even less help when it gets down to the management. It is universally sparse and tends to be contradictory. Medicine feels that exercise is necessary and instigates physiotherapy; a few talk about 'rest', whatever that is; some even suggest sleep therapy; and the majority say that there is no treatment, or that nothing can be done. The sufferer is not unreasonably confused and depressed.

Research is going on, and in the last couple of years or so has undoubtedly increased, but it is still mainly directed towards viruses, muscle disease, immunological aspects and not so much towards developing rational management programmes, an approach that I believe is the most effective. Work is also needed to look into the epidemiology of the problem, (the way in which it starts and its causes).

My understanding of what might be going on in the disease process of AOPVFS took a very large 'U turn' in November of 1989. In chapter nine of the first edition of my book, I suggest that there is a significant 'power producing problem' within the skeletal muscle. I am now not at all sure if that is actually true. The evidence for significant skeletal muscle disease causing fatigue is lacking, indeed there is some to the contrary. Let us now go through some of the various points that I made at that time and the new information that is available now.

It appears that the greatest area of conflict from the sufferer's point of view seems to be medicine's stance of 'Psychiatric' versus 'Organic', to question the concept of whether the disease process actually exists. Once you have transcended that position and believe that there is a disorder called M.E., the argument continues with 'central' versus 'peripheral'. I shall have to tell you what central and peripheral means.

Central

Any kind of dysfunction, disorder, or disease that affects the brain and the spinal cord.

Peripheral

The rest, all the bits and pieces outside the brain and the spinal cord are peripheral.

There are many symptoms that suggest that there are significant central problems. The big question is whether there is actually anything wrong at all with the muscles or the body, or any other organs for that matter, and if so, what? The reason for looking at muscle is that firstly there is a lot of it, and you can get to it fairly easily. Pinching bits of muscle from people is not very difficult. Stealing bits of brain from patients does not go down too well, so for the meantime we are going to have to stick to muscles. Secondly, there are lots of symptoms that appear to be directly related to muscle – weakness, fatiguability and pains, which seem to suggest that there is something wrong.

The muscles

Weakness

If you are a sufferer it is apparent that there are symptoms that would appear to be localised to muscle – the muscles of the limbs appear to be weak, they do not seem to have the strength that used to be there. In the past when I have examined a patient I felt that I could detect a degree of true muscular weakness, especially if examining the patient after they had done some physical activity such as climbing the stairs or walking on a treadmill. The degree of weakness observed by a doctor is by asking the patient to grip one's fingers or to offer some restriction whilst the patient raises a leg, bends a knee, or moves the toes. The doctor then judges whether for that patient's sex, size and build, there is any weakness. I felt that patients with AOPVFS could produce a near normal degree of strength when encouraged and that if there was any weakness it was not particularly significant. Certainly the degree would not be on the same scale as one might expect to find in other neurological diseases. You can appreciate this kind of clinical assessment is often far from accurate or convincing, as muscle strength is really a measurement and a reflection of the patient's co-operation. I am not suggesting that the patient is deliberately unco-operative but if they are feeling unwell and generally fatigued this will be reflected in their inability to produce a maximum force. Muscle power is thus dependent upon the functioning of the brain. Furthermore, I have seen, and I know of other doctors who express the fact that some patients just are not able to give of their best when they are examined and in these situations there is deemed to be a great deal of psychological 'overlay', which means that the problem lies in the mental approach of the patient!

There are ways around this limited clinical assessment and hospital laboratories have developed ways of assessing muscle power and muscle fatigue, which I will discuss later but in principle, this is done by direct muscle stimulation and takes away the 'brain input'. They are very specialised laboratories and are not readily available.

Muscle Wasting

Muscle wasting does occur, but it is a sign of clinical mismanagement, and one of the consequences of '*over resting*'. Do too little for too long and the muscles disappear. This situation is actually quite easily tested by using single fibre EMG studies and muscle biopsy which will show the specific changes that occur in muscle during wasting, of type 1 fibre atrophy and reduction in mitochondrial concentrations.

In patients that are not over rested or manage their disease correctly, muscle wasting does not occur. There will of course be a loss of fitness and there may be a loss of muscle bulk, but muscle biopsy and electrical studies are not significantly different from those of normal people.

During the clinical examination, any muscle problem, be it fatiguability or possible weakness, must be seen to be global, occurring in all muscles symmetrically, just as much on the right as on the left, and on the top as on the bottom. One must not be able to be in a position to show that the problem is limited to one arm or one leg as opposed to the other. Any 'true' localising weakness of this nature would bring into serious doubt the diagnosis of either AOPVFS or M.E. Any kind of lesion like this must be associated with another organic neurological disease process such as polio, multiple sclerosis, neuritis or the like.

Myalgia

The complaint of polymyalgia (widespread muscle pain) especially after effort is common and seems to be one of the more convincing symptoms suggestive of a localised muscle disorder. Some patients' muscles certainly are painful, others' are not so, expressing more of a leadened feeling, as though they have been dragged through six feet of mud with wellington boots on or have run a marathon race when they have in fact actually only walked 100 yards. Some have a dull ache or tenderness when touched or squeezed, a soreness, a burning. Various qualities are expressed, but still the majority point to the muscles and say they hurt. The discomfort is more severe immediately after activity, tends to be localised to the muscles used and gradually eases, becoming uncomfortable overnight and causing restlessness, keeping the sufferer awake, and disturbing sleep, thus increasing the general fatigue the next day.

Muscle Twitches

Not only do the muscles that are used in physical activity ache and feel fatigued but they frequently 'twitch'. Patients express the feeling as though there is something in the muscles crawling about, they feel alive, on the move, shaky, tremulous, jumpy, after activity.

Tender Spots

Apart from global muscle aching one can often find muscle pain in very specific tender spots, small areas about the size of a 1p or 2p piece. They tend to vary in position and intensity, coming and going, quite often in very short periods of time, occurring in one muscle one day and possibly another muscle the next.

Muscle Pain in Stress

Myalgia can be seen to occur after mental activity such as reading, studying or stress. It is widespread and much less frequently seen than that which occurs after physical activity.

True Muscle Disease

If the myalgia is severe a possible pathological process affecting muscle should be considered that may not be part of AOPVFS or M.E. Myalgia occurs in rheumatoid arthritis, thyroid disease, metabolic processes and many other diseases. Myalgia should therefore be appropriately investigated, and should always include a muscle biopsy and single fibre EMG studies.

Muscular Fatiguability

The symptom of muscle fatiguability is the mainstay of the diagnosis. It is *always* present, it is said to be 'pathognomonic'. Without it the diagnosis of M.E. or AOPVFS is untenable and cannot be made. It is the symptom of increasing inability to perform the physical activity required. Weakness is defined as a failure to generate force and fatigue as the failure to sustain it. Sufferers find that if they do not do much their symptoms are minimised, especially the muscle fatigue: as activity increases so does fatigue and work output begins to diminish. Patients find that they pace themselves to their level of illness. When severely affected life becomes a simple potter. The sufferer quickly becomes conditioned to his or her level of physical capability but hopefully as the condition improves and the degree of fatiguability diminishes the work and power output increases. But at any one moment during the illness, if there is a sudden increase in physical activity, the patient suffers for it. Doing something makes them tired and fatigued and there is usually a commensurate increase in their other symptoms. For things to improve there is a required period of rest.

The degree of fatigue to which the patient suffers depends not only on their degree of illness but also on the speed, rapidity and degree of physical activity undertaken. As an example, if a patient has a degree of illness that allows them to struggle over a 100 yard walk in a time of say five minutes, then the patient's muscle fatigue would be very much worse if they tried to do the 100 yards in one and a half minutes. Equally the patient would suffer in a similar, if not identical fashion, if they tried to do 150 yards at the same rate as they would do the initial 100. So it is, the amount and the rate at which physical activity is undertaken that governs the degree of fatigue suffered.

These various symptoms of muscle fatigue, aches and pains, twitching and movements not unreasonably add up to the suggestion that there is something 'severely wrong in the muscle'. If there is something wrong in the skeletal muscle there may be something wrong with the heart muscle giving rise to the palpitations, missed beats, dropped beats, etc., that are all too common and frequently very worrying to the patient who often asks if they could suffer a heart attack or something similar. The muscle of the gut might be involved, explaining the symptoms of indigestion and irritable bowel syndrome. Visual focusing problems may also originate in an underlying muscle problem, as also could be the possible explanation of the arteries and veins (which also contain muscle) being involved causing the blanching of the face, cold hands and feet, flushing etc. All of this muscle dysfunction could have a peripheral origin.

The central component to muscular fatiguability

There are observations that suggest that at least some of the muscle symptoms are generated by a central component. As mentioned in the paragraph on myalgia, I have seen patients who would complain of an increase in muscle aches and pains if they do a lot of mental activity. It does not seem reasonable to suggest that this symptom would be generated by a muscle problem, more likely when the brain is goaded into action, that there would be some kind of increased neurological output to the muscle and this would in some way develop an increase in muscle pain. There is in fact a complex nerve system that conveys messages from the muscles back to the central nervous system and vice versa, that could be involved in the development of such muscle pain.

Whilst an increase in mental activity is not common in the generation of myalgia, a symptom that is almost universal amongst sufferers is that they find that their muscle energy output diminishes with increased mental stress and strain in what appears to be a linear fashion. A little bit of mental activity that is paced appears not to have too much of an effect, but as the mental output is increased the patient not only tires mentally but also physically. The more the mental activity, the greater apparent muscle fatigue and reduction in physical output capability. This symptom is best explained by a central cause. Likewise, the complaint of sudden draining and loss of energy. Patients note that when they are mentally, but more usually physically, active they can experience a sudden draining of energy, disappearing as though someone has pulled a plug out of their feet. They become weak and wobbly, and have to sit down. It is remarkable that observers can also detect this as there also appears to be a loss of colour from the face, which becomes grey and pasty. I cannot see how all the muscles in the body could suddenly lose their strength for any reason other than the loss of central drive, where the brain output regulating the system has failed. Some find that if they eat food when they are 'weak', especially something sweet or sugary like a Mars or chocolate bar they have a sudden surge in strength. This can occur to such great effect that patients find themselves eating more food, more frequently than necessary, with a resulting increase in weight. There has been a suggestion that this symptom is due to hypoglycaemia or altered glucose metabolism, although whenever patients' bloods are tested their blood sugar and metabolism is normal.

In the acute phases of the disorder the degree of weakness and fatigue varies very rapidly, in some cases hour to hour. It would be difficult to see this caused by a peripherally based muscle disorder.

Centrally generated symptoms

There are a large number of symptoms which could not be argued in any other way than being purely centrally generated. Psychological symptoms of anxiety, depression, the central fatigue experienced after mental activity, loss of concentration and memory, the sleep disturbance, etc. These account for 50% of the problems for most sufferers but the ratio between central and those that appear to be peripherally based varies from one person to another. How these central symptoms are generated, what causes them, and what maintains them are important questions and I think that it is going to be a long time before we get the answers. As we are not in the position of being able to open somebody's brain up to have a look and see what is going on, we cannot yet get to the biochemical level necessary to study the disease process in the brain. X-rays, Computerized Axilal Tomography, Electrical Studies with EEG's or detailed Magnetic Scans using Magnetic Resonance Imaging (MRI) are all not detailed enough. There is a new system in America called P.E.T. scanning which may well be helpful, as it looks more at the functioning side of the central nervous system, studying blood flow and the uptake of oxygen within the brain during mental activity.

All of the central symptoms are functional, not structural. There is *no* evidence that the brain is damaged in any way. Post Mortem studies cannot help as you cannot see memory or depression in a dead brain so we are going to require other kinds of neurological studies to help understand the problems that lie in the central nervous system.

Returning to the question of whether there is a peripheral muscle disorder or not, let us first look at what we know to tell us what sort of disorder we may expect or not expect to find.

If you look at the natural course of events in AOPVFS, the first thing that one would expect to find is a disorder that affects the brain and the muscles in a very similar fashion. Equally the disease must be similar in heart, lungs, the gastro-intestinal system, eye, bladder etc. The process has to be variable from person to person and within that same person, from one time to another, and when as usually occurs, the patient gets better, there must be no residual effect. Those that do recover can do so completely so we cannot be looking at a clinical picture of a destructive disorder, or a permanent disease of the central nervous system or muscle as they are not capable of regenerating themselves but leave scars. Also conventional investigations already available such as Electro-Myogrammes (EMGs), MRI Scans, Muscle Biopsies etc. would have shown some kind of permanent lesion before now and none is known to occur (with the exception of a paper published in 1985, Ref.1). The disease is non-inflammatory, functional and reversible. This sort of problem must have an answer that lies at a subcellular level within cells, with the biochemistry, or abnormal transmission of molecules or chemicals either through the brain, muscle or blood. The disorder is one where the body is not working properly and suffers a biochemical dysfunction.

Let us look at some of the abnormalities that have been demonstrated and that have been published. Let me straight away say that I am not sure that these various abnormalities and findings can be necessarily applied to my own patients with M.E. and AOPVFS, because my tight criteria may not be applicable to the other groups studied. This is probably an unreasonable supposition, because there must be some considerable degree of overlap, as researchers now agree on the clinical subsets and it is likely that we are looking at similar, if not identical patients.

Dr Peter O. Behan is Professor of Neurology at the Institute of Neurological Sciences at the Southern General Hospital, Glasgow, and a leading expert in the field of M.E. He and his wife Wilhelmina, a pathologist, and Dr Eleanor Bell from the Enterovirus Reference Laboratory in Scotland produced a paper entitled, 'The Post Viral Fatigue Syndrome, an analysis of the findings in 50 cases'. It was published in the Journal of Infection in 1985 (Reference 1).

The patients studied were eighteen men and thirty-two women with ages ranging from 17 to 55 years, with an illness lasting from three months to twenty-two years, with a mean duration of five years. The cases he described gave a 'clear cut history of a viral or viral like illness as the initial event'. All the patients were examined and were shown to have 'no abnormal clinical signs'. A series of routine investigations including blood count, biochemistry, muscle enzymes, X-rays etc. were performed including Single Fibre EMG studies, published separately (see below). Phosphate nuclear magnetic resonance studies were done on six cases in a laboratory located in Oxford, the Director of which was Dr George Radda, and one case finding was published (see below). In summary the paper describes a whole series of abnormalities, 70% were found to have impaired lymphocyte function of the T cells, depressed in a similar fashion found to be present in other types of viral illness, cancers and auto-immune disorders. There was an impression that there was a high incidence of Atopy (allergic disease). A large number showed autoantibodies and there was an association drawn between the Post Viral Syndrome studied and the finding of high antibody responses to Coxsackie B viruses.

The main thrust of the paper however were findings that suggested specific muscle disease. The patients when exercised, showed 'gross weakness' afterwards and it was suggested that the muscle aches and pains and fatigue were associated with the various specific muscle findings then described. Muscle biopsies done on the patients showed that 75% of the biopsies demonstrated scattered muscle fibre necrosis, in other words, specific muscle destruction. These findings were suggested as being 'subtle' but 'definite' and predominantly affecting type II fibres. Further electron microscopic appearances of muscle described 'bizarre tubular structures' and 'increased peripheral mitochondria'. The tubular structures appeared to be mainly associated with the cases with myalgia. The paper suggests that the 'muscle appeared to bear the brunt of the disease' and this was further supported by a paper later published on Single Fibre EMG studies (see below) and by 'metabolic changes noted during NMR studies'. The paper concluded that 'these findings confirm the organic nature of the disease' and that 'a metabolic disorder caused by persistent virus infection and associated with defective immuno regulation is suggested as the pathogenic mechanism'.

This is of course an important paper describing peripheral skeletal muscle abnormalities and changes that would support a diagnosis of muscle disease as the cause for or at least the major part of the patient's problems. Reference in the paper was also made to the central fatigue seen in their cases.

From the description of the patients studied it must be concluded that they closely resemble those of AOPVFS as studied by myself.

The single fibre EMG studies

To increase your understanding of the published work I will tell you what Single Fibre EMG Studies entail. The commonest muscles studied are those of the back of the arm and as you probably know muscles are stimulated electrically via nerves.

A needle with an exceptionally small point is placed between two muscle fibres, care being taken not to damage either. This is done by very gentle manipulation until a pair of fibres are found that are being stimulated by the same single nerve fibre (one nerve fibre in the arm commonly stimulates upwards of 200–300 fibres, so it is not that difficult). The fibres are activated by asking the patient to lift a finger, and the electrical impulse passes down the muscle fibre and is recorded as an electrical action potential passing the tip of the needle. The time that it takes for this action potential to travel along the muscle fibre and pass by the tip of the needle varies a little bit, so the action potential might alter by a few milliseconds in front of or behind the action potential travelling down the other muscle fibre, and the time interval between these two potentials can vary, one being faster and the other being slower, so the action potential appears to 'move', backwards and forwards in time. This is termed 'Jitter'. In normal healthy people this jitter has fixed limits. If the limits are exceeded then they are said to have a 'pathological jitter value'. This is seen in several disease processes affecting nerves and muscle, diabetes and cervical spondylosis for instance. So an abnormal finding is not pathologically confined to one disease but its presence has been seen in Post Viral Fatigue Syndrome where it has been suggested to represent an abnormality of the muscle fibre cell membrane and the rate at which it conducts electrical stimulation and supports a metabolic muscle disease.

In 1985 (Reference 2) Goran A. Jamal and Stigg Hanson published a short report on Single Fibre EMG studies done in forty cases of Post Viral Fatigue Syndrome. They were the cases referred to in Behan's paper discussed above. 75 per cent of these patients demonstrated 'pathological jitter values' in a large number of fibres.

With this demonstration of abnormal electro-neurophysiology affecting the membranes of skeletal muscle fibres there was further evidence to support a peripheral fatigue. Yet more fuel to this fire was added with a paper published from the Oxford Centre for Phosphate Nuclear Magnetic Resonance (Reference 3). One patient with prolonged Post Viral Exhaustion (one of Professor Behan's patients) was studied by this very complex investigation which showed that the muscle fatigue produced during exercise was accompanied by early intracellular acidoses and there was speculation that the defect occurred in the oxidation process of muscle energy provision. This is a convincing demonstration of a peripheral muscle metabolic problem.

All of these papers show specific muscle abnormalities, certainly sufficient to answer the question as to whether there is any evidence to support peripheral fatigue in muscle. I knew all of this in 1985–86 and as a result I wrote chapter 9 entitled the Musculoskeletal Problem and came to the conclusion that there must be something terribly wrong. It would have been easy to have continued to believe that this was the case, that at last we were beginning to get to understand more about the nature of the development of the fatigue but this has not proven to be so.

Shortly after finishing the manuscript for the first edition of *Understanding M.E.* a paper was published from Liverpool (Reference 4) from the Muscle Research Centre and it made some very controversial points with regard to the Management of M.E. and Chronic Fatigue Syndromes, suggesting that there was *'no peripheral muscular fatigue'*. I made some generalised enquiries and was told, without exception, that the head of the Muscle Research Centre at Liverpool University was a respected international expert, Professor Richard Edwards. The problem with the paper was that it was not really clear as to whether the patients studied did in fact qualify as having Post Viral Fatigue Syndrome, as was suggested. It simply said that some of the patients studied had had a 'history of a viral infection shortly before or at the onset of their symptoms'. The major problem has always been, and still is, to define precisely what you are looking at so that all experiments and papers can have confidence in uniformity. I was not at all sure that this paper applied to AOPVFS, but because of its importance and conclusions I decided that I had better go and see for myself, so in the summer of 1989 I went to Liverpool to discuss the various points with Professor Edwards. I stayed for several days and my most important terms of reference were to establish the type of patient studied and to assess in my own mind whether the experiments were appropriate to the measurement of fatigue in those patients. I was totally satisfied on both counts.

Whilst finding that the majority of patients studied fulfilled the looser definition of my own criteria for M.E. there were certainly some who clearly had the clinical condition of AOPVFS. The only point that I would make was that the majority of the latter had had their illness for some considerable time, certainly in excess of two years. However, that does not appear to present any significant barrier. I then went on to learn how these patients were assessed.

In brief, the patient had a history taken, examination, lots of blood tests and then they were placed into a specially designed physiological chair where their right leg would be used for the experiment. It was bent at the knee to 90° in a comfortable sitting position and the ankle was attached by a strap to a force strain gauge. The patient would be encouraged to try to straighten the knee as hard and as long as they could, while many measurements were made then the patient's muscles in the thigh were stimulated electrically to a maximum contraction.

Measurements were again made and blood tests taken. Shortly after a period of recovery, about one hour, the patient was exercised on a bicycle and they were made to pedal until they felt exhausted and then the measurements in the chair were repeated all over again. By this time of course, the patient was feeling fatigued but that was not the end of it. The whole process was repeated in exactly the same fashion the following day when the patient's fatigue was worse. The experimental procedure was again repeated in its entirety three days later when the patients again were expressing fatigue to say the least, 'death's door' some said! These studies revealed however that these patients' muscles worked *normally* throughout the days of the experiment. They could produce a maximum force on their own account and also reproduce that maximal force in a totally normal way when their muscles were stimulated and made to work for them. So whatever else was wrong there was very clearly nothing wrong with the 'power production'.

I took many opportunities to have some further discussions with Professor Edwards about M.E. in general and I asked him what relevance he felt the various abnormal findings that had been published had to play in the concept of muscle disease. He thought they had very little. He referred me back to paper (Reference 5). He suggests that a 'vicious circle' of biochemical change is responsible for the perpetuation of the muscle symptoms in M.E. and that it is caused by a low habitual activity. The argument here is circular, a virus infection at the beginning produces a temporary enzyme defect, mental depression, lots of symptoms and inactivity. The inactivity leads to a decreased content of mitochondria in muscle. This leads to exercise intolerance. Which leads to muscle pain and to further inactivity.

I concur with this particular statement, this has been the experience that I have drawn in trying to understand how patients with Post Viral Syndrome who stay in bed for five weeks, ever manage to get better and I have written a chapter on that elsewhere ('Why is Rest so Bad').

Waggonmaker et al go on further to suggest that the abnormalities demonstrated by Arnold when investigating a patient with Post Viral Fatigue Syndrome by Phosphate Nuclear Magnetic Refinance is literally what you would expect to find in somebody who was under activated. They say 'although it was suggested that this was due to some kind of disorder of metabolic regulation we wish to indicate that it may be entirely due to a low concentration of mitochondria in the muscle of this patient'. Waggonmaker et al also continue to point out that when patients decrease their activity habitually there are changes in the type of fibre that occur in the muscle and that one will develop an early acid production at very low levels of activity and this early acidosis may be responsible for myalgia. In all, Waggonmaker and his co-authors show that severe changes occur in the muscle during prolonged inactivity that lead to the perpetuation of severe symptoms and in the discussion of the paper they state that 'the M.E. Association is publishing substantial amounts of information on the 'disease' and its advice to patients is to rest as much as possible. We wish to point out, however, that the low content of mitochondria in the majority of these patients may indicate that they need therapeutic exercise' and continue 'these patients also appear to suggest that trials of therapeutic exercise may be worthwhile in patients who present you with pain and exercise intolerance because of metabolic defect and without a definite underlying cause (effort syndromes and post viral fatigue syndromes) therapeutic exercise could possibly improve both the physical and the mental well-being of these patients'.

It all boils down to a very simple sentence: virus causes immobility, immobility causes immobility, causes immobility . . .

My whole concept of the muscle disease had been smashed. The primary executive function of muscle is to produce power. It does nothing else and in these very convincing experiments I had had it demonstrated to me that patients with AOPVFS had no peripheral fatigue. This being the case what relevance do all of these demonstrable muscle abnormalities have in AOPVFS and M.E.? Well, whatever they have, they do not have any effect on power production, so whether they are pathological and whether they have any significant role to play in the pathogenics of this disease is therefore brought into serious question. Various further publications appeared during 1988 and 1989 on muscle function. Lloyd et al (Reference 6) produced a paper coming to exactly the same conclusions as Waggonmaker's. In this case they were using the upper limb instead of a leg, and there was no demonstration of any reduction in force. However the patient group studied here were suffering from 'a fatigue syndrome' that had no criteria for an active viral type start to their illness, so what was being studied would be very difficult to identify.

In June of 1988 (Reference 7) some muscle biopsies were sent down to the Charing Cross Hospital from Professor Behan in Glasgow, on patients suffering from M.E. Studies showed that some 30 per cent had enterovirus RNA inside their muscle tissue. Later, other patients in the same group were shown to have Epstein Barr Virus particles inside skeletal muscle biopsies. The amounts of enterovirus RNA was really quite high and I subsequently met Dr Len Archard, a recognized expert in the field, to discuss their relevance. He was of the opinion that enterovirus RNA inside skeletal muscle would have to have a significant impact on the metabolism of that tissue and he would have thought that there would almost certainly be a reduction in power output. In 1989 he along with others (Reference 8) later showed that these enterovirus RNA sequences were in fact genetic mutations, that they had for the first time shown a basis for persistence of enterovirus infection inside skeletal muscle tissue.

I thought at this stage that it was time to try to clarify precisely where this fatigue is and to see whether these apparently opposing views could be drawn together. I had a whole lot of muscle biopsies left over from the original studies that I had done a year or so ago and I asked Dr Archard whether he would be kind enough to look at these for enterovirus sequences. Out of one hundred and forty samples looked at, only one had enterovirus inside the tissue. An enormous difference from those seen from Glasgow. I sent the same biopsy material to Glasgow for microscopic examination and we did not find the fibre necrosis or mitochondrial abnormality that were seen in Professor Behan's paper of 1985 (information to be published).

I sent thirty or so patients with AOPVFS for further neurological studies to look at their Single Fibre EMG assays and *not one* of them had the abnormality of jitter so I thought that yet again, the only possible answer must come from the fact that we are looking at totally different groups of patients and/or that there is 'a lot more enterovirus in Glasgow!'. Most of my patients come from the southern half of England. This latter suggestion becomes a possibility when one looks at a very recent publication (Reference 9). Here, when looking at antibodies both IgG and IgM in patients with Post Viral Fatigue Syndrome and in normal controls there were found to be very high levels, 24 per cent or so positive in both the patients and the controls. This suggests that 24 per cent or more of the population of that area of Scotland has had a recent enterovirus infection.

We need to be able to resolve conclusively the question as to whether there is any peripheral muscular fatigue. Several papers certainly suggest pathological abnormalities in skeletal muscle, but do these have an effect on fatigue peripherally? Edwards says No!

The answer really is quite clear. What we must do in the near future is to take a group of patients with a clear clinical diagnosis, that all parties would accept, and I would suggest that of AOPVFS: further, that this group be yet more highly refined, that they have evidence of a recent enterovirus infection as seen by positive IgM antiviral antibody or evidence of a persistent enterovirus infection with a positive VP1 – possibly both! and that the skeletal muscle biopsies should demonstrate enterovirus RNA sequences and that this group of patients are looked at by the Liverpool team and their muscle fatiguability or function assessed. This will give us a definitive answer.

Let us assume, for argument's sake, that there is indeed no peripheral muscular fatigue, that the problem is centrally generated and the muscle fatigue is perceived and not actual. Is there any way in which these various muscle abnormalities and findings can be drawn together and a sensible logical reason for them given? I think so.

There is good evidence for a persistent enterovirus infection, in some cases a persistently positive IgM response to the enteroviruses, VP1 positive assays and most convincingly, evidence for persistent mutation of enterovirus sequences in skeletal muscle biopsies. The abnormal muscle histology, appears to be slight and possibly as little as only 1 per cent of muscle fibres are involved with persistent enterovirus infection (work to be published). So, if one argues that the other 99 per cent are not affected and are working normally, then one would not expect to see any reduction in muscle power output as it is incapable of detection experimentally. One per cent of affected or infected muscle fibres however could be enough to cause the myalgia and would limit the patient's physical activity. If the enterovirus infection of the muscle cells is very short lived and fleeting, going from one fibre or group of fibres then to another, this could explain the migratory tender muscle spots and as there is no permanent damage done to the muscle fibre during this self limiting mutant infection, they would be expected to fully recover, thus not leaving any kind of permanent scarring. This does not however answer the question as to where the seat of disease is.

So where is this disorder and what is it, what is causing it and what maintains it? There is little doubt, from what I have told you that the fundamental problem must lie inside the brain. There are blood tests that show virus, muscle biopsies that show virus and in other situations virus components and elements can be detected and there is no doubt that this 'virus' is there. It is likely that there is no fatigue in the muscles and the viruses that are there are in such small quantities that they are unlikely doing very much pathologically speaking. The more you look at the various bodily peripheral symptoms in this disorder, the less one is convinced that there is anything structurally wrong elsewhere. The various heart symptoms are not stained by any kind of heart disease and when the patient gets better those symptoms go away. There is no abnormality to find on ECG. The same goes for the blood vessels. There is nothing actually wrong that causes the cold hands and feet. The abdominal symptoms of indigestion, bloatedness, irritable bowel syndrome, again do not appear to be due to any kind of pathological abnormality. The blurring of vision has encouraged many patients to go to the optician, who cannot find anything wrong.

Looking at these symptoms they appear to be functional. Whatever bit is causing problems, is not working properly. But there is nothing wrong with it; it is the central control mechanism in the brain that seems to have gone wrong.

So we are looking for an area of the brain that could give us all of these symptoms if affected, and there is one. It is called the Hypothalamus.

There is a universal law that says if there is a simple answer to a complex problem and a complex answer to a complex problem, the simple answer is always right. A simple answer to the question, where is this disease? is the hypothalamus. I am not going to give you an entire anatomical and physiological lecture on the hypothalamus but it is the hub of the brain. It lies between your ears, behind your eyes, at the base of the brain in the middle. It is a route directory. In computer hardware terms, it is the mother board. In functional terms, it is D.O.S. The hypothalamus is the area that instigates all of the automatic body function operations, the autonomic nervous system. The vagus nerve, which originates here, controls heart rate, blood pressure, blood vessel diameter and any functional abnormality at this level could answer your palpitations, cold hands and feet. The rest of the vagus nerve goes down into the abdomen, and is responsible for the gastro-intestinal system, movement and secretion of juices. An abnormality in vagal function here could cause irritable bowel syndrome. The hypothalamus has lots of 'centres', controlling such things as temperature, sweating, breathing eating etc. There is no doubt that a functional disorder of the hypothalamus in this disease could answer the generation of every symptom complained of peripherally. Can it also answer the abnormalities of central higher function problems? Yes, it can do that as well. It roots the areas of the brain that are responsible for wakefulness or sleep, emotion, depression and anxiety. It is at the crossroads of the highways that are responsible for thought processing and memory. There may of course be other areas of the brain involved and there probably are. You cannot have such a large and important structure like the hypothalamus being involved without disorganising virtually every other part of the brain's function and capability.

This is a theoretical concept, a working model. I think that to theorise a hypothalamic dysfunction is the easiest and simplest way to answer every problem and symptom of AOPVFS and M.E. If this is the case, we will need to develop investigative capabilities to test the theory and in some research centres there are such capabilities being developed and the results are promising.

What maintains this disease?

Presumably a virus, but this may not be true. A large number of patients have evidence supporting a persistent virus infection of one kind or another and it may well be that the functional hypothalamic disorder is maintained by that virus. I presume that when people get better this persistent virus infection goes away. Otherwise of course it would knock that theory on the head but another explanation might be possible. *We all get* Post Viral Fatigue Syndrome. If I get an enterovirus infection I am ill for a few days or a week and get better but during those few days I have the symptoms of Post Viral Fatigue Syndrome that others continue, unfortunately, to suffer from for the next few years possibly. The seat of infection in these patients may well be their intermittent persistent sore throat. This source of infection, for some reason, is not cleared, virus particles are pushed into the blood stream and go into the muscle and there is no reason to suppose that there is not the same kind of persistent virus infection in the central nervous system where it causes the functional disorder in the hypothalamus. It may be that this persistent infection in the throat gives rise to other means of maintaining the hypothalamic dysfunction. There may be as a result an abnormal production of chemicals, substances capable of producing the flu-like symptoms, for instance, interferon, interleukin and others, some of which we probably do not even know about. These complex substances could cause an abnormal central nervous system dysfunction and maintain the disease.

There are a large number of patients in whom no matter how often we do the various blood tests, we cannot find a virus, so is their disorder maintained by a virus?

Why not? Because you can't test for it in the blood, it does not mean to say it does not exist. The problem lies in the central nervous system. Who knows what capabilities the virus has of producing persistent infections within the central nervous system and you would have to start looking at the brain directly for evidence of this. Why do a blood test? Why do a muscle biopsy when the problem lies in the brain? You do not do a blood test for multiple sclerosis, you do not do a blood test for a brain tumour; you do the appropriate neurological investigations and I suggest that the appropriate neurological investigations for M.E. have not yet been developed.

Apart from those that have a persistent virus maintaining their disorder, which I accept is highly likely, there are of course many other possible explanations. The one I favour is the capability of the hypothalamus to develop some kind of dysfunction precipitated by a virus but not necessarily maintained by it. Many functions in the brain, including the hypothalamus, work on a negative feed-back system. As an example of this we can look at the mechanism that controls eating. There are a collection of nerve cells in the hypothalamus that are stimulated when you are hungry. You eat something and there are a collection of nerve cells and receptors in the stomach that tell you when you are full. There are chemical detectors which have a similar action and these structures will pass messages back to the brain saying that you are full up and have eaten enough. The brain then reduces its drive to eat. Similar negative feed-back systems are behind the control of such things as breathing, blood pressure, temperature regulation and most hormone control.

Let us suggest that our sufferer gets an initial enterovirus infection which is not adequately cleared because of an inappropriate or ineffective immunological response because the patient is under stress. As a result a persistent enterovirus infection develops in the central nervous system, and the hypothalamus in particular. This persistent infection could last for a few weeks and set up an imbalance, a loss of the regulatory control of these various feed-back systems so that the regulation is pushed over in one direction or another. When the persistent virus infection settles, or goes away, these systems are not actually capable of returning to normal regulation, they become permanently upset, their thermostat is set on high or low.

So we have a virusly precipitated hypothalamic dysfunction that if maintained by the virus for a few weeks or so, has the capability of producing a permanent dysfunction. One that can slowly recover if handled correctly and that for reasons that we do not understand, if mismanaged, can lead to a permanent irrevocable disease process and a functional disorder of the central nervous system that seems to be irretrievable. If whatever dysfunction occurs in the hypothalamus lasts for more than two years or so it reduces the chances of getting better and if that dysfunction lasts five years there seems little capability of recovery.

Predisposing factors in the development of AOPVFS

During my initial involvement with AOPVFS I noted that when I asked the patients to recount what happened right at the beginning of their disease most volunteered the information that they were under stress at the time. As there are many causes of stress it was not practical to explore this area fully in the questionnaire, so most of my information is drawn from experience. However, to provide some kind of numerical back-up, questions were included as to whether the patient had suffered stress from an emotional, mental, occupational, financial, medical or bereavement source or from chemical exposure. Forty-three people responded that for a period of time prior to their disease process they had been under pressure that was unusual for them. The time over which that pressure had been applied was quite variable, but six to nine months was not at all uncommon, and it is a feature that I continue to notice as the most likely contributor among all the other possible factors.

Taking these possible associations one at a time, the first would be:

Work: Sixty per cent said that they had been working particularly hard, with either extra hours or extra pressures being put upon them, for at least a year. It did not come out that this type of stress was physical; no patients claimed that they were having to dig more holes in the road, or bake more buns. The pressures appeared to be more those of added responsibilities and mounting problems, leading to an increase in mental stress (see below).

Emotional: Forty-three per cent said that they were emotionally stressed from relationship problems with their partners. This was often to be found in conjunction with work problems.

Mental: Eighty-five per cent admitted they were under mental stress for the reasons mentioned above and below. Usually this stress manifested itself in anxiety problems, tenseness, irritability, argumentativeness, an inability to relax, sleep disturbance, a lowering of mood, enthusiasm and drive and, not uncommonly, depression. These symptoms were to be found over extended periods of time.

Financial: Five per cent suggested significant financial problems, although subsequent to the study the incidence of this seems to have decreased.

Medical: I believe that various medical strains and stresses are involved in the pathogenesis of both AOPVFS and slow onset M.E., although I cannot give figures here. By virtue of my very specific disease definition, the patient with AOPVFS must have been perfectly fit and well until the time of the onset of their disease, so people with any other medical problems would necessarily have been excluded from the questionnaire. However, I have heard several stories that make me suggest that medical stress is probably a significant feature.

In the last few years, several women have said that during the course of their confinement, or around the time of the delivery of their baby, they developed acute temperature and malaise from which they did not recover. The attending physicians always suggested that it was something to do with either a urine or womb infection, and there was never any convincing evidence that it was a virus – but it is a possibility to bear in mind.

Other stories involve people suffering accidents – one woman who had fallen off a ladder and broken her leg developed an acute fever and malaise while in the hospital having it set. Two patients developed an acute illness and failure to recover in a typical post viral story after a gall bladder and hernia operation respectively, while a further patient suffered an acute fever and malaise after having her bladder investigated with a telescope. Slow onset M.E. symptomatology can be found subsequent to the same type of medical strains.

Bereavement: This was put into the questionnaire because bereavement had been a significant problem in one patient, but in the study, and indeed subsequently, it did not arise again.

Chemical exposure: None of the patients that I was studying suggested that they had been acutely exposed to any chemical that they could remember in the previous few months. None were particularly keen gardeners using abnormal amounts of pesticide, and none volunteered any environmental possibilities.

Some of the factors above have been implicated in the possible development of disease and, while I appreciate that stress factors are extremely common these days and are related to a lot of other medical problems, it was something that I felt gave a very strong 'push' to the development of AOPVFS. When looking at the slow onset type chronic stresses are very difficult to interpret, because they would have to be present for a long period of time in order to justify the gradual onset of disease.

It is also worth noting that if stress is particularly marked in the development of these disease processes, it must also cause further difficulties in the diagnosis. Stress carries the additional symptomatology of anxiety and depression which, coupled with the subsequent depressive symptoms that are so closely tied with AOPVFS, induce the physician to make a psychiatric diagnosis.

The psychiatric symptomatology found in AOPVFS and M.E.

This is a very important aspect of the disease, as in many cases these symptoms are the most severe and disabling that the patient experiences yet at the same time they can be some of the most accessible to treatment and disease management.

In a number of severe illnesses there is an increased expression of pre-morbid psychological traits. This means that a person who was psychologically well-balanced before the disorder would not suffer intense psychiatric problems subsequent to it; but a person who was depressive would find this exaggerated. Of course the exception proves the rule, and there are no doubt a number of people who would be described not only by themselves, but also by their physician and family, as being mentally very stable, yet who after the development of their disease become severely psychologically disturbed.

It is certainly true that in any significant disease there is at least a small, and usually a large, component of interplay between psychological and physical symptomatology. Physicians feel that you cannot have one without the other, and this is nowhere more evident than in AOPVFS and M.E., where defining the physical symptoms is extremely hard. All are subjective, and have no markers; for example, is fatigue a result of psychological or physical symptoms? Anxiety, depression and tiredness, even the aches and pains and sleep disturbance, can be argued on a basis of psychological symptomatology, rather than a physical one, and that has been the direction the medical profession has taken for a number of years. However, I believe that the vast majority of psychiatric symptomatology is based on organic brain disease, that the virus or viral effect alters synaptic transmission and thus brain function so that psychological symptoms are produced as a result.

It is interesting to compare those who have ΛOPVFS and are immediately supported by their physician on this basis with those who have consistently been told there is nothing wrong with them physically, and that it is 'all in the mind'. Patients in the former group have a good understanding of their illness and are not usually on any medication for psychological problems, whereas the latter group tend to be on antidepressants and/or other drugs and have probably seen psychiatrists. The psychological symptoms in the supported group are much less disabling than in the other, so it is evident that medical understanding of the disorder in the first place lessens the psychiatric morbidity in AOPVFS.

The symptomatology

Neurotic

Anxiety: This is a major symptom which is found in 90 per cent of cases, tending to occur in the early stages and diminish as the disease progresses. Patients express feelings of inner tension, nervousness and unwarranted apprehension that something disastrous is going to transpire. This leads to agitation, irritability, and often arguments in the family.

Phobias: Phobias are irrational fears and it is quite common for patients to develop these, becoming nervous of going into public places, large shopping halls, pubs, etc. This probably stems not only from anxiety, but also from the fact that patients often cannot deal easily with noise and crowds.

Panic attacks: Seen as an extension of the first two symptoms, full-blown panic attacks are not uncommon. Anxiety builds up, probably in a crowded public place where the phobic symptomatology comes into play, and a full phobic attack develops, with sweats, increased agitation and palpitations, leading to overt panic.

These panic attacks can also occur in situations which are normally less stressful, such as at work or even at home.

Affective symptoms

Disturbance of mood: Another very common finding is a marked emotional lability. The patient can be reasonably well, yet suddenly be overwhelmed with tears for no reason at all. Cross words from a colleague or a member of the family, films, TV programmes, and even the news on TV or radio can cause extreme distress. This can lead to phobic traits, in that the patient will not listen to the news, watch the television, or even read a newspaper, because of the emotional stress caused.

Such outbursts of tears are rapidly followed by tension, nervousness, aggression and anger.

Loss of drive and enthusiasm: Some 60 per cent of patients find that they just do not have the will to do things any more; not only do they lack the physical energy, but they experience the loss of mental drive.

Primary depression: Also seen early in the disorder, but tending not to diminish as is the case with anxiety, depression, in conjunction with lowering of mood and drive, can be a crippling problem. It tends to vary during the day, often being quite severe first thing in the morning, easing in the middle of the day, then returning later in the evening. This problem can be very severe, so much so that there appears to be no light at the end of the tunnel, and the feeling that health will never return has on occasions led to suicide. (I have not myself had a patient who has subsequently committed suicide, but I have seen three cases where attempts have been made.)

Secondary depression: This is sometimes difficult to differentiate from the primary depression, which is the depression that is actually part of the disease. Secondary depression is reactive and its incidence depends much more on the patient's pre-morbid personality. Of course, it is not unreasonable to find people feeling deeply depressed about the fact that they are very unwell.

Sleep disturbance

Many patients find difficulty in getting to sleep; they feel that their brain is still 'switched on' and despite being absolutely exhausted they remain wakeful. When they do finally drop off they only sleep fitfully and wake up in the morning as tired as they were when they went to bed. This undoubtedly compounds the problem, as a good sleep pattern is of paramount importance.

Psychotic symptoms

I include this heading merely to express my observations that psychotic symptoms are not associated with M.E. or AOPVFS. I have not found patients having unreasonable beliefs or delusions, hearing voices, seeing things, being thought-disordered, or suffering from paranoia. In looking at well over a thousand cases, I have met one person who after the development of their disease became acutely paranoid, believing that people were saying malicious things about her, but this one case would reflect statistically the amount of severe psychotic illness seen in the general population. I am therefore quite certain that one does not develop psychotic illnesses such as schizophrenia or manic depression as a result of AOPVFS or M.E.

Organic brain syndrome

Concentration: The majority of patients complain that their concentration is badly affected. They suffer not only difficulties in grasping information but also in disseminating it, which mars their writing and speech. They express the feeling that they know what they should be doing, but cannot muster the necessary thought processes to take logical action.

Taking these functions individually, writing problems include an inability to get the correct word from the brain down on to paper, and spelling, handwriting, punctuation and grammar deteriorate. Difficulties in reading are expressed as a problem with getting the words from the paper into the brain – while the patients can read the words, by the end of the page they cannot remember what it was they read, and so are forced to go back and reread the text over and over again. Some find that their concentration is initially quite good, but rapidly falls off as they tire. In severe cases, some give up reading altogether.

As to speech, difficulties include finding a conversation with even one person tiring, while discussion with two or more people leads to problems in collating changes in thought direction. Patients will sometimes mispronounce words but more commonly they are simply unable to find the right one; they may even lose their entire train of thought.

Visual concentration: Many patients find that they cannot understand a storyline on the television because they have difficulty in following the sequence of events. They then tend to stop watching as further sensory input produces tiredness and irritation.

Memory: Memory goes hand in hand with concentration and the two are difficult to differentiate. Patients forget simple things that they had always been able to remember in the past – recipes, names and addresses, telephone numbers, something that was said to them five minutes beforehand tend to disappear. They have very little problem with long-term memory; it is the everyday trivia that causes the most difficulty. Many patients find that they have to write things down immediately in order to reduce this problem. Some who are in a position to do so have learned to have a secretary always present to do their remembering for them.

Other higher brain problems: Generally speaking, those who have to use their brain power for their work find their capabilities as reduced as those who have to use their muscles. The ability to be able to produce complex mental steps and thought processes is most affected and difficulty in even visualizing a problem, let alone being able to think it through, is common.

Just as with the muscles, overuse of brain power has a 'knock-on effect' in that if a little bit too much mental output is required day by day, the ability to be able to produce that output slowly diminishes and increasing anxiety, depressive symptomatology and sleep disturbance patterns set in. So the symptoms and problems exactly parallel the physical ones, but not necessarily in exactly the same degree – I have noticed that in some patients the physical incapability is extremely marked, where their psychological and organic brain function is not so severe, and vice versa.

It is when the psychological symptoms are profound that one finds a higher proportion of primary psychiatric diagnosis, rather than where the physical symptoms are more clearly demarcated.

Temperature in AOPVFS and M.E.

The normal temperature, as measured by a clinical thermometer under the tongue, should read 98.4°F/37°C, although one must bear in mind that a lot of people constantly show a slightly higher or lower reading which is normal for that individual.

The majority of people do not appreciate what their normal temperature is, since the only time they ever take it is when they feel ill, with the exception of women who are trying to become pregnant and take their temperature every day so that they can see when they ovulate. Every woman has quite a marked variation in temperature throughout her cycle, even within one day, and there are many things that can give rise to a slightly raised temperature apart from an infection; this should be borne in mind when considering the temperature in relation to M.E. and AOPVFS.

In the cases of M.E. that I have studied, I have found no significant abnormality in temperature. In AOPVFS, however, there are some quite interesting abnormalities; in the initial flu-like illness there is usually quite a marked rise in temperature, a recorded level of 102/103°F/40°C being not at all uncommon. This begins to fall and then, within a week or so, despite the fact that a lot of people feel flu-like, hot and cold and sweaty, the temperature reads as subnormal. This finding is extremely consistent, and can be several degrees Fahrenheit or at least one degree Centigrade below normal values. The more unwell the patient the lower the temperature, and as the patient begins to recover the temperature returns to normal.

I have not seen any patients who have had a significant rise in temperature during the later course of their illness; indeed, if such were the case, I would say that it would indicate some other factor. This is a means of establishing the difference between an acute new infection and an exacerbation; a high temperature would be a sign

of a new flu or cold, while a normal one would point to a recurrence
of old symptoms.

Post viral syndrome in children

There is no doubt that fatigue syndromes occur in children. I am
going to draw a line at the age of sixteen when discussing the
various problems. As a child becomes a more mature adolescent
they are much more able to communicate their own symptoms and
feelings to take control of their own disease process and understand
the consequences of it. In young children the parents are the ones
that 'feel' and control the illness. Also one must appreciate that the
various investigations, particularly those of the virological 'tests',
are much more easy to interpret and more reliable in a sufferer
over the age of sixteen. As you will see later, interpretation of
the virology under the age of sixteen is much less dependable. The
younger the patient the more difficult it is to understand the nature
of the illness. I have no doubt that AOPVFS occurs in children
but there are even more doctors working with children who do
not believe it exists than there are adult physicians who believe
in AOPVFS. I accept however that the subsequent illness that
follows a virus infection in children is more likely to be influenced
by phychological factors and have less of an 'organic' nature than
in the adult process. The reason for saying this is simply that the
illness of AOPVFS and indeed any other illness in a child, is really
not the property of the child but mainly shaped by the influence
of parental attitudes especially in the very early acute phases.

By illustration we will take little Johnny, once more, he gets
an acute viral illness and whether or not he actually goes to the
doctor in the first few days or week or so does not depend upon
Johnny but his Mother and Father, probably more upon Mother.
Johnny will be taken to the doctor sooner rather than later by
a worrying or possibly over-concerned parent. Alternatively the
parents might feel that it is simply a virus and he does not need
an antibiotic or any specific remedy and the child is encouraged
to stay at home.

After the expected recovery doesn't start to occur after one week or whatever the child is taken to the doctor, the history of the illness will suggest a virus infection and the doctor will probably confirm that, saying that it is some kind of 'flu', or glandular infection and that it will settle down with no specific treatment. Now the whole process depends upon the parents interpretation of their child's symptoms. They see a continuing fatigue syndrome with or without the majority of all the symptoms mentioned elsewhere. They keep going back to the doctor, no obvious reason is put forward other than the fact that he should recover in due course and when this does not happen it depends entirely upon the doctor's understanding of Post Viral Syndrome in children as to what happens next. The parents see an ill child, the doctor may not. If the parents are very anxious further investigations may be instigated by insistence, probably a Consultant Paediatric opinion will be sought and again the diagnosis depends upon the physician attending. Even though AOPVFS is much more readily diagnosed in the 1990s than it was before, there is still a very large body of paediatric opinion that does not believe that it exists or that treat it with a great deal of caution or more often scepticism. Alternative explanations are rapidly sought and it is much more easy to elicit other possible reasons for the child's continuing illness than it may be in the adult: school refusal, sibling rivalry, over protective parents, child behavioural problems being the more common suggestions sported by the medical profession. It is because the illness is not controlled by the child but by the relationship of the parents with the medical profession that lead to the consequences that I so frequently come across. The majority of AOPVFS in children is unremarkable and even though the child might not become well for several weeks or even months, with support and understanding about AOPVFS from the medical profession the illness abates uneventfully. If one gets, as one does quite early in this situation, polarised attitudes then the consequent problems arise. The 'ill' child is seen to be ill by the parents. They present their 'ill' child to the medical profession who may be very sceptical and say that there is actually nothing wrong. The parents are bemused and uncertain and so of course will be the child who may be feeling very unwell and the whole family, being told that there is nothing wrong, start to behave in unpredictable fashions. Children play up, become difficult, sleep disturbance starts, eating disorders occur, children might struggle back to school with relapsing symptoms. The parents may continue to push the child or take a reverse stand and start to over protect. Behavioural problems occur in the child and to a greater or lesser extent in the parents as well. It is at this stage that the problem is at its most serious and difficult. Protracted illnesses start to occur, parents continue to encourage the child to remain unwell, not purposely, but they see their child being 'ill' and by keeping the child off school. This rubs off on the child who continues to be perplexed and looking up at their parents, behave accordingly. Looking at it from the child's point of view it must also be very difficult, if not impossible to understand what is going on. They have an illness from which they have not recovered, they feel 'ill' and they are clearly confused and perplexed about the lack of understanding. Their parents are probably taking either an over-protective stand and encouraging them to rest or they are being difficult from the child's point of view in that they are forcing them to go to school when they are not feeling well. The child therefore knows that there is something wrong with them, otherwise why should they either be put to bed or why should they be sent to school when they feel so ill. Clearly they can see the problem is not understood, the parents are not confident in their handling of the situation and prevaricate. They may also find conflicting feelings, one week understanding and sympathy and the next week an aggressive 'let's get on with life' type of approach. Equally the child must be aware of the fact that the doctors clearly do not understand what is going on. It is therefore not at all surprising that behavioural problems and emotional difficulties occur.

All of the above comments apply to AOPVFS. The waters get deeper and even more muddied when it comes on to the slower onset M.E. or Chronic Fatigue Syndrome in children where there is no evidence of an acute viral start.

To diagnose M.E. in the adult, I look for a good pre morbid personality and health prior to this Slow onset Fatigue Syndrome. If you have a child being presented by the parents having been unwell since they were a baby or an infant and they had lots of other problems like sleep disturbance, feeding, colic etc. the interpretation I suggest is impossible. So once again I have drawn a line for myself and said that any child with a fatigue syndrome under the age of seven must be cared for by a Consultant Paediatrician and a diagnosis of M.E. or AOPVFS is untenable. I would *never* make a diagnosis of Acute onset Post Viral Syndrome of a child under the age of seven. I would go further and say that a non specific M.E. Syndrome without an acute viral start is untenable under the age of sixteen.

The chances of developing an AOPVFS are about one in a thousand. Whilst it is perfectly possible for an entire family to go down with the same virus infection the chances of two members of that family developing AOPVFS are really quite small, certainly a lot greater than one in a thousand. I have seen very occasionally two members of the same family developing AOPVFS at the same time and presumptively and historically from the same 'virus'. However the chances of developing two people in the same family at totally different times with different viruses I believe is extremely remote, greater than one in a million, especially as we have shown that there is no genetic predisposing factor. In other words, 'it doesn't run in the genes' or 'the blood' for people to develop the illness.

If therefore you have one adult in the family with M.E. or any other kind of fatigue syndrome then it is going to be very unusual for a child to go down with a virus and get a Post Viral Syndrome. However, I am aware that whilst this statistically would be about one in a million I have seen a great number and I believe that the majority of those are psychologically based. It is also more than likely the case that both are psychiatrically based if two children or more get Post Viral Fatigue Syndrome at differing times in the same family.

Management of M.E. in Children

With a few refinements, the management of the disease process is very much along the lines seen in adults, but as already suggested the disease is under the continuing guidance of the parents. One needs to be very sure of the diagnosis which is entirely clinical. *No* positive tests must be sought, with the sole exception of specific EBV serology. With the correct disease management recovery is the rule. It is even more important in children than the adult to have co-operative and understanding medical support, the hub of which should be the General Practitioner. I am constantly phoned or written to by parents asking if I can help them make their General Practitioner understand, that the General Practitioner and the Consultant are unhelpful, that they do not believe in M.E. and Post Viral Fatigue Syndrome. There is nothing I can ever add to the advice that you must always take your General Practitioner's guidance and help. I cannot suggest a conflicting opinion. I believe in the 'organic' understanding of Post Viral Syndromes of their various types. Your doctor may not, that does not make him wrong or me right, but if you see the whole situation getting worse and your child's illness becoming more extended and things generally going downhill, then ask for a further opinion. Do not be afraid to put forward a measured sensible approach. On the assumption that you are getting helpful medical advice regular visits to the doctor are suggested because it is so often seen that if a lot of external advice is taken patients tend not to be regularly followed up and can in fact get lost and entrench themselves in what may be inappropriate therapeutic regimes by 'doing their own thing'. I mean by this, to avoid some of the more strange alternative therapies and explanations. The General Practitioner should be *in control* of the disease process and hopefully take some of the major directioning and conduction away from the parents, who can then be seen as instruments, rather than dictators, of how to get better. Children are more likely to work with parents, who are being themselves told precisely what to do, rather than if the parent becomes the sole orchestrator.

As pyschological problems are prevalent in ill children, a constant careful monitoring should be applied looking for depression, anxiety, rebellion, and behavioural problems. A child psychiatrist may be very appropriate here, if a psychiatrist is not available then a psychologist would be an essential member of the recovery programme. The illness should be openly discussed between all of the members of this team without fear or favour and as near as possible a well balanced approach achieved. It does not help to polarise views into the 'Organic' versus 'Psychiatric'. Parents should be ever mindful of the psychological problems that occur in children just as much as the physicians should be aware of the organic. Modified activity programmes are the main stay to recovery and should of course be kept to as near as possible, but children hate to be regimented and an occasional break with a reward for being good is also very helpful. Antidepressants are probably less easy to use in children than they are in adults. Side effects are difficult to control, and I am not trying to produce a whole herd of zombie like patients. Many of the new antidepressants have not been passed for the use in children and for this reason alone the therapies and combinations of drugs that may be helpful, especially in the acute phases, should be controlled and prescribed by the consultant psychiatrist. As in the adult, these medications are used to improve sleep patterns, to restore meaningful and rewarding rest during the night, to maximise physical and mental activities during the day. They are very helpful in modifying depressive and anxiety symptoms, upsets and temper tantrums.

The problem of education

Children are constantly pressured into getting back to school. Education is something that they require and need and it is the County's duty to ensure that they do. A short term AOPFVS illness does not seem to cause problems, as long as the child suffering has complete medical agreement and back up, education does not suffer. Subsequent problems lie in three areas:- firstly, is the patient and family who find themselves at continuing odds with their medical advisers.

Second, those that are improving and are well enough to go back to school and how this should be attained.

Third, what education can be provided for those children that are severely afflicted and affected by Post Viral Fatigue Syndrome?

The first problem occurs after a variable period of time and is something that I try to help patients avoid at all cost. If, because of polarised attitudes, there is a breakdown in the relationship between medicine and the parent and the consequent loss of the child's treatment, medicine will tend to leave the child alone for a period of time. That situation cannot continue and as long as the child is under age, medicine has the capability of advising the powers that be that something will have to be done. This takes many forms, one of these is that the parents will eventually find themselves in a Court of Law and the child made a Ward of Court. They can actually take the child away from the family home into care or the court can say that this child will go back to school. Whether the child is actually well enough or not depends upon the medical advice and from the several cases of this type that I have seen, there is no doubt that the child at this stage is ill and probably not from the AOPVFS which may have started the whole thing off. Failing to respond has led to a dichotomy of opinion, as I have intimated earlier. By this time the child has developed behavioural problems or hysterical conversion syndromes with psychosomatic symptoms like abdominal pains, shortness of breath, headaches, panic attacks and even paralysis. Wheelchair or bed bound, the child's horrendous situation continues to confirm to the patient's relatives that it is physically ill. By now, alas, the situation confirms to the medical profession, quite rightly by this time, that the child is psychiatrically disturbed.

I would like to see this scenario disappear and I think that with the sort of co-operation between medicine and parents, that I have suggested above, there is no reason why children should end up in this position. It is usually the education authorities, on doctor's advice, that 'nothing is physically wrong', that instigate court procedures after the child has not been back to school. After the initial virus infection by say two or three months, enquiries are made, the doctors say that there is no reason why the child should not have education and the education inspectors start knocking at the door.

The second problem dealing with the child that is recovering, is getting good medical support with understanding parents on how the schooling is to be resumed. Application of a modified activity programme is needed. It is not a good idea simply to get a child out of bed one day and put them back to full time education the next. Excessive, mental and physical activity makes symptoms worse. Schooling is mainly a mental activity and initial return to school should be gentle and slow, perhaps one or two half days per week over a period of a month or so, so that improvement is monitored. Return to school should initially exclude physical education activities. As the child becomes more confident and able to retain information during class the lessons should be increased and when full-time has been reached over a period of possibly several months, then the physical educational programme can be re-started again in a slow measured fashion. Whilst I appreciate that education is one of the most important things that young children can have, all work and no play makes Jack a dull boy, and I would advise that rehabilitation programmes should include a few visits to the cinema or various rewards to encourage the normality of life for the afflicted child. A positive dynamic encouraging approach should always be sought. Children frequently get depressed and low, or simply fed up with lack of progress; and this in its own right can produce deleterious effects and backward steps. Bear in mind that supervision by a third party is always advisable, ideally a psychologist or counsellor, to make sure that both the parents and the child are handling the disease process to the best of their ability, that either are not trying to go forward too fast or too slow. Exacerbation should be avoided as this prolongs the disease process.

The third problem is looking at the child that is ill for a longer period of time, unable to manage the physical journey to school and not making the progress that is hoped. Here, the problems are not just that of loss of education but loss of normal life. Children are supposed to have friends, peer groups and experience the rough and tumble of life and the ill child of six months or one year's standing loses this, so they should be provided where at all possible. Where school is physically a long way away, it may be appropriate that transport be provided enabling the child to get to school earlier in their illness rather than later, but if that is still too much one must consider the capability of providing home tuition. This is something that should only be looked upon as being necessary after a long deliberation. The provision of home tuition of course takes away some of the need to recover and get back to normality. Some doctors, certainly those who tend to disbelieve the whole concept of M.E., would say that provision of home tuition is forbidden, that it simply compounds the illness, not only for the patient but also the parent and takes away all drive to recovery. I would argue that as long as it is given after due care and attention, that home tuition is needed, necessary and desirable. Home tuition is a one to one relationship and a smaller period of time is required to get across an amount of education, and the amount provided should be small to start with and should be gauged upon the patient's mental capability. Having established the programme the amount of tuition can be increased as the patient improves. There is a maximum amount of home tuition that is provided by the Education Authority and the amount varies very much from one authority to another. Having established a routine one must remember that illness must not be made to be comfortable. You may say that is unfair, and would never happen but I have seen it occur many times, as home education is easier than getting up and going to school, especially on a cold dark morning. The home environment can become a padded palace, and the whole process might become just too easy. I have yet to find one child, or indeed one adult, that doesn't seem to have an intimate knowledge of TV soaps.

I have been involved with many of the doctors in Great Britain in developing a further understanding of M.E. and AOPVFS. I thought that we had begun to make inroads into getting physicians to take a more open view about it. Unfortunately that continues not to be the case, especially relating to children. There are few paediatricians who believe in Post Viral Syndrome or M.E. Herein lies the danger. As an adult you can always walk away from a piece of medical advice and ultimately the responsibility is your own. That is not the case in child medicine.

If you go to a doctor who is too polarised in one particular direction or another, then you can end up with a child that is iller than he or she should have been.

If the doctor you see has a very strong physical view of M.E., then you may find yourself missing the psychological and psychiatric problems that may be there or that may develop.

If when seeking an opinion you get dismissive medical advice you will find that you cannot simply get rid of it. It is not so easy to get a second opinion, or another alternative view. If medicine believes that there is nothing wrong with your child or that you are being over protective or a totally unreasonable parent, then it can apply sanctions and will. I have met many Consultant Paediatricians who are adamant that M.E. does not occur in children, and who believe that the entire M.E. Syndrome is created in the child by the parents. Apart from individual beliefs or disbeliefs there are occasionally statements which indicate a particular line held by a body of opinion.

An example of such, the Royal Society produced a briefing document in September of 1990, and whilst it does specifically say that the document does not 'constitute a statement of policy by the Royal Society or by the Association of British Science Writers' there is a small section given over to Chronic Fatigue in children. There was not any suggestion that there was a condition called Post Viral Syndrome or M.E. that may have an organic basis. The author described the disease as typically being some kind of behavioural or psychological problem and again here is seen the advice that it is 'important not to arrange for a home tutor which will simply reinforce and prolong the problem. Getting them back to school as soon as possible, remedying the cause where possible. Equally it is important not to perform tests which simply make the parent think there is something wrong with the child.'

I cannot believe that there is simply no such disease as Post Viral Fatigue Syndrome in children or that various types of M.E. just do not exist and I cannot accept that style of approach that infers that it is all in the mind. Where psychological problems, abnormal behavioural patterns, both from the child and the parent can be seen they should be handled positively, openly and with care, but I know that I have seen children in whom that sort of explanation just simply cannot stand up and when such a dismissive approach is adopted the problem is compounded.

EBV and children

This virus is mainly associated with glandular fever, a disease that is usually found at and around sixteen years of age, and from which only 10 per cent of us suffer. Why that is, nobody knows. However, since 92 per cent of us have been exposed to the Epstein Barr virus by the time we are twenty, most of us have had a virtually subclinical disease of which we would never have been aware without the availability of assessment of antiviral antibodies.

The Paul Bunnell and heterophile antibody tests appear to be less reliable in diagnosing a primary EBV infection than I once thought, and I believe that many people who are told that they have glandular fever are not suffering from primary EBV. In any event, the younger the child, the less likelihood there is that they have ever had an EBV infection, and, so far, I have no evidence to demonstrate that there can be a reactivated state in children. As this is found in adults there must be an age at which it comes into play, but it is as yet undetermined.

Enteroviruses in children

The enteroviruses are extremely common in children; they usually cause a summer flu between late May and September, most notably in six and seven year olds. Antibody assessment looking at enterovirus IgM shows that 70 per cent of children have evidence for a recent enterovirus infection. These results are on the whole quite sustained and it would not be at all uncommon to find an enterovirus IgM response lasting for six to nine months, although three months is more usual. Consequently, the interpretation of this antibody response becomes impossible when trying to apply it to AOPVFS, let alone M.E.

I suspect that in this age group, and probably in older children, the VPI test is also uninterpretable. I think that we are going to have to look much harder at the assessment of VPI antigen viraemia in a larger control population of children before we can say with any degree of certainty that this test can be applied to them.

In children over the age of seven the presence of enterovirus antibody diminishes so that by the age of twelve something in the region of 5 per cent give a positive result. By the age of sixteen or seventeen, less than 1 per cent of any control group show an IgM response.

Another point that must be borne in mind is the marked geographical variation in enterovirus responses. For instance, several studies in mid and north Scotland suggest that the incidence of enterovirus infections is up to three times greater than in southern England and in some control groups and in some years the studies demonstrate very high proportions of positive IgM responses.

My final conclusion, therefore, is that the VPI test and an enterovirus IgM should not be applied under the age of sixteen until we have more information about their interpretation.

Other viruses in children

I have not, as yet, come across a child in whom another virus can be implicated in M.E. or AOPVFS, although I have seen four adults in whom shingles has been associated with the AOPVFS syndrome, shingles being a reactivated form of chickenpox. I have not encountered any type of post viral syndrome as the result of chickenpox, or indeed any of the other common childhood virus illnesses such as German measles, mumps, etc.

The virology in the whole child group is impossible to interpret at the moment, and the diagnosis of AOPVFS must be entirely clinical. The definition of M.E. as I perceive it is that of a slow onset persistent enterovirus infection, and as this relies upon a positive VPI test it cannot apply to children at present. The slow onset fatigue syndromes that do affect children remain quite uninterpretable, both clinically and virologically, and the arguments about how and why they occur therefore remain open to intense debate.

The disease in children is complicated by three factors: the continuing disbelief of the medical profession; the close involvement of the parents; and the immature personality and the dependency of the child suffering from the disease. The incidence of depression and fear in children with any kind of long-term illness is well established, and if that child is presented to the medical profession by a parent who believes that the illness is entirely physical only to be met by doctors who are not in concordance with this, then arguments break out, the child becomes more confused, and the whole family becomes isolated. In extreme cases, of which I have seen several, the social services become involved and a care order may be put on the child on the grounds that the parents are unfit. So what should be done to avoid this?

My own feeling is that every child with a possible acute onset post viral syndrome or any other fatigue syndrome should be assessed and cared for, using a multi-disciplinary approach, involving not only the parents and their GP but also the school, social services and child psychiatrists and psychologists. All of the people involved should have a working understanding of M.E. in all its forms, and accept a possible organic basis for it while being ever mindful of the psychological components that are bound to be present.

It is difficult enough to gauge the amount of exercise versus rest that is required by the adult, this being a subjective matter, and it is clearly undesirable to allow a child to be in control of this without supervision. Again, a team approach must be sought.

The irritable bowel syndrome

Some of the more major symptoms that occur in AOPVFS and M.E. are typical of classical irritable bowel syndrome. There is still a good deal of discussion within the medical profession as to the definition of irritable bowel syndrome, but the common view is that it is a functional disorder of the whole of the gastro-intestinal tract – from the oesophagus down including the stomach itself, small intestine and large bowel – where there is no structural or anatomical lesion such as an ulcer or a tumour that could explain this dysfunction. It is usually caused by a hypermobility of part or all of the bowel, which gives rise to a set of variable symptoms.

The bowel is a tube which varies in diameter, the largest part being the stomach which, when full, constitutes quite a large container. This empties into the small intestine, which resembles very flexible, slightly dilatable hose pipe some 4.5 metres (15 feet) long, emptying into the large bowel. The latter varies quite a lot in size, depending upon how full it is, but it is usually somewhere between 2.5 and 5 centimetres (1 and 2 inches) in diameter. The whole of the bowel is covered in a membrane which to a greater or lesser extent limits its dilatory capacity, and the walls of the intestine are made of muscles that are variably arranged around and along the bowel. These muscles cause constriction down the tube from the stomach to the small bowel, and into the large bowel, forcing food to travel through the gastro-intestinal system.

The lining of the bowel varies, but on the whole it is a uniform mucous membrane. It has a variety of functions which include producing enzymes to help digestion and containing cells to absorb the digested food, while other cells are specifically designed to soak up water and nutrients and to form faeces. When food reaches the stomach it remains there for probably two to four hours, during which time it has enzymes and acid poured on it. The acid kills bacteria and most viruses and the enzymes start the digestive process, so that by the time it leaves the stomach the food is simply a thin, homogenous, soup-like mixture to which bile from the liver and enzymes from the pancreas and small upper bowel are then added.

Digestion starts in the stomach and continues through into the upper parts of the small bowel. By the time it has been in the small bowel for four to six hours food is beginning to be absorbed, the majority of food absorption taking place in the lower small bowel, an area called the jejunum. The food takes somewhere in the region of twelve to fifteen hours to pass through the small bowel, still as a very thin watery liquid out of which most of the useful substances – food, minerals and vitamins – have been taken, and this thin liquid is then squirted into the beginning of the colon, which starts in the lower part of the pelvis just on your right-hand side, at around the level of the hip. The function of the colon is to take water, electrolytes (potassium, sodium etc.) out of this mixture and leave you with a solid, excretable lump of faeces. The colon is thus responsible for maintaining water balance.

The symptoms of irritable bowel syndrome include intermittent abdominal pains, 'indigestion' in the upper part of the stomach just underneath the ribs, probably coming on quite quickly after eating, and pains associated with the small bowel, which tend to be in the centre of the abdomen, just around the navel. These can be quite sharp and colicky, whereas the classical symptoms of colonic pain are low, windy, longer colic pains just above the pubis. Pains associated with irritable bowel can be in any or all of these areas and they come and go – they may not be there for a few days, they may be there for weeks on end.

These abdominal pains are often associated with the feeling of being bloated and uncomfortable, and are usually accompanied by some degree of intermittent large bowel dysfunction with diarrhoea and/or constipation. The patient experiences a rumbling, as if the whole lot were constantly on the move more than usual, and also, especially in AOPVFS, a feeling of nausea.

It is not unusual to find an associated symptom called 'hurry'. This is when your stomach seems to start working immediately you eat or drink something and you have to go to the toilet. Some people envisage this as their food 'going straight through them', but it in fact represents a peristaltic stimulation where the intake of food or liquid initiates an over-active bowel movement with consequent emptying at the rectal end.

It is not uncommon to find patients with AOPVFS going to their doctor complaining of these various abdominal symptoms. While the patient is often told immediately that it is irritable bowel, neither doctor nor patient will probably be satisfied until tests such as a barium meal, barium enema, and fibro-optic examinations are undertaken. It would not be unusual to find a small hiatus hernia, which may, incorrectly, be given as the explanation to the problem, but otherwise one would not expect to find a structural abnormality that could explain the symptomatology. So what causes it?

The accepted medical view is that the commonest cause is anxiety, which results in over-activity of the nerves that control the gastro-intestinal system. Virtually the whole of the function of the gastro-intestinal tract is controlled by one large nerve called the vagus nerve, which originates in the base of the brain, travels down as a thick, cord-like structure through the chest and into the stomach, divides up thousands of times into small intricate nervous pathways, and provides a calming effect on the bowel. The stimulating effect to the bowel and its hyperactivity depends upon the sympathetic nerve supply, another automotive nerve stimulation.

The normal bowel function is an intricate balance between these two nervous systems. Upset this balance for one reason or another and you either end up with severe constipation from under-mobility or an irritable bowel from over-stimulation.

Suggestions as to the causative agents of irritable bowel syndrome in AOPVFS and M.E. patients include food allergies, candida and viruses in the gut. I am not sure that any one of those explanations is sufficient. AOPVFS is a functional disorder that is seem to affect the central nervous system and the skeletal muscle, and I see no reason why the same dysfunction should not occur within the control of the gastro-intestinal system. However, I have noticed that certain foods contribute significantly to the irritable bowel syndrome seen in AOPVFS.

The treatment of the irritable bowel syndrome as seen in AOPVFS and M.E.

Traditional medical advice: This mostly consists of dietary advice, which would be to substantially increase fibre intake. Antispasmodics are usually suggested, but other than that most areas of medicine seem to be quite unhelpful.

An anti-candida regime: If you believe that candida has anything to contribute, then follow an anti-candida diet and take a course of Nystatin or other anti-candida remedies.

Food exclusion diets: I recommend these highly as I have found them very helpful. They consist of reducing one's diet to a few basic foodstuffs and then gradually reintroducing other foods to find those that cause trouble (see pp. 224–25). I also favour adding one or all of the following:

Charcoal Activated charcoal is just what it sounds like – bits of semi-burnt wood. Young willow charcoal can be bought as tablets not much bigger than a polo mint. Chew about half a dozen of these a day and swallow them with some water for a harmless, non-medicinal remedy.

Charcoal has one remarkable property: it is very good at absorbing gas. This has been well-known for a number of years, and it is used in other situations as a biological gas filter. It is capable not only of removing some of the gases found in the grumbling flatulence that irritable bowel syndrome causes but also some of the more unpleasant smelly gases.

Peppermint An old-fashioned remedy which was almost thrown out of my prescribing list when I graduated, but is certainly coming back again. It is a powerful anti-spasmodic, stopping griping pains and aiding normal bowel peristaltic movement.

Antidepressants One of the side-effects of antidepressants, the quadracyclic type especially, is that of dampening down hypermobility within the bowel and helping to restore normal function.

High fibre intake When you have established what foods you can and cannot eat without upsetting your bowel, find ones that are on the high fibre list and eat a little more of them. High fibre intake is essential for healthy bowel activity.

There are no specific rules for following any of the above suggestions, bar taking the prescribed dose of antidepressants. Simply experiment until you find what brings relief.

9
THE NATURAL HISTORY
OF AOPVFS

I have seen in the region of 3,000 patients, mainly those suffering from AOPVFS but certainly many complaining of the slow onset M.E. disorder. When discussing the history at the first interview, the most important part is to find out how this condition started. This can be difficult because memory is limited and sometimes when patients have been ill for a couple of years or so they cannot remember everything that has happened. However, I have always been impressed by the fact that even after this time patients can recall the day, even the date that they developed this apparently devastating 'flu-like' illness and some of the events that lead up to it or perhaps it is not so surprising as many have had their lives ruined from that day. Thus I have access to an enormous amount of historical information, predisposing factors, time of year, age of onset, sex predisposition, and many other bits of information. Subsequent discussion with the patient will allow analysis of the clinical course of their illness and of what factors make patients better and recover, why others might get worse and stay ill. Developing computer programmes to help answer questions are easy these days and I have had several software packages made for my database and these enable me to analyse large numbers of patient information in a very short period of time and this can be enormously helpful. I have found quite frequently that facts tend to be the same or similar each time and this begins to mean a great deal.

My first problem was how to go about measuring the disorder. The numerous symptoms, whilst often similar, can be very variable and the clinical course fluctuates. With statistical analysis it became clear that there was nearly always an underlying trend for patients with AOPVFS to get better and those with the slower onset M.E. not to, and they appeared to have different disease processes. I have not continued to use the questionnaire that was developed earlier (see chapter – 'The Study') as since that time I have found that it is not important to discuss individual symptoms or problems that patients complain of. When a person is ill all the symptoms are worse; when they get better the symptoms improve, so a collective look at the complaints is adequate. Indeed it does not help to single out a particular symptom or to treat it individually.

AOPVFS is assessed on purely clinical grounds. There are no tests, parameters or markers. The blood tests that we have available at present have no quantitative value and they appear to have no prognostic influence. Whether there is an enterovirus, a reactivation of EBV, primary EBV or no viral abnormality demonstrable at all, does not seem to make any difference to the clinical progress in either AOPVFS or M.E. So how do we develop a method of looking at the clinical progress and being able to help with the understanding of how recovery might occur and when that might happen? These are all questions that are extremely important to the sufferer to know and for the doctor to be able to answer.

The way that I chose was to take the patient's functional capability. If you add up all the symptoms, they are going to prevent that person from functioning normally. It still appears that the dysfunction suffered is divisible into mental and physical aspects but I take an overall view and ask how much these various symptoms are interfering with that patient's normal life. This would give me a scale of capability of function. If you took this and plotted against time, then you will have a graphic representation of how that patient is recovering in functional terms. In the graph drawn in Fig. 16, the vertical axis represents the degree of fitness/function, the bottom of which reads 100 per cent well (this might be the equivalent to somebody who was as fit as an Olympic athlete and few of us are that well). Assuming that we have average health,

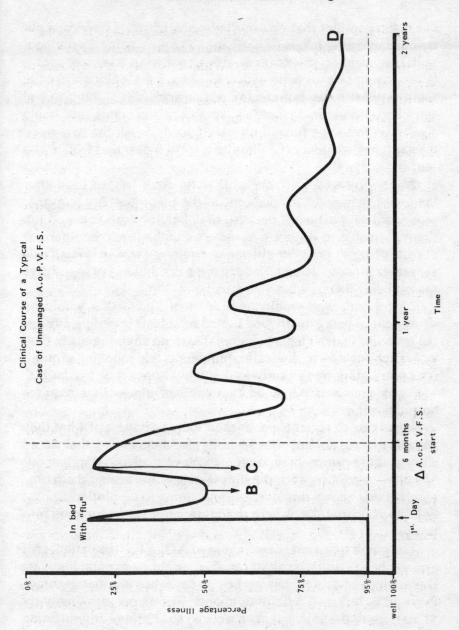

Fig 16. Clinical course of a typical case of unmanaged AOPVFS

one might consider that we are all 95 per cent well. I have then put in four increasing levels of ill health. The first being 75 per cent well; this might represent being able to participate in most events in life, being able to cope with a full-time job, looking after the children, family etc. but missing out on social life. Going to bed early because of the symptoms, resting at weekends, not being able to go to the pictures, entertain friends, wash the car, weed the garden or whatever. Certainly a level of illness that would stop sporting activity.

50 per cent well would be able to do one's job, or look after the house, home etc. 50 per cent of the time, possibly requiring occasional days off work because of ill health, flexi-time and job sharing, unable to do one's housework without needing periods of rest, being 50 per cent efficient, requiring extra help such as a gardener, window cleaner, daily home-help, and a very supportive spouse being half of what you were.

25 per cent well would be a level of illness that would be equivalent to being nearly bed bound or at least spending most of the time sitting in a chair, being unable to do anything other than look after one's own physical requirements and lounging around, not contributing significantly to the family support or needs.

0 per cent well might be that level of illness that requires hospitalisation.

By talking to patients about their daily activities, of what they are able to do or not do, one can easily give them a score that would allow you to position them on the graph vertical axis. Finding out how they have been since the illness started and seeing them on a regular basis allows this level of functioning to be plotted against time, the horizontal axis here in Fig. 16 being seen to extend into two years.

The graph is of a case of unmanaged AOPVFS, the patient is of average health until the arrow marked on the horizontal line, '1st Day', which indicates that particular day when the patient finds themself in bed with a 'flu-like' illness. The arrow marking point 'B' represents partial recovery a week or so later, but still suffering from mild flu-like symptoms the patient has tried to return to work or manage the household duties only to find a return of their symptoms causing a relapse at point 'C'. The illness has now run into six months represented by the vertical dotted line at which time the diagnosis of AOPVFS can be made (by definition). It is hoped in the future that this diagnosis will be made earlier and the vertical dotted line moved towards the left.

It is during these first few months of the acute phase that the symptoms are at their most florid. They show a marked degree of fluctuation both in severity and variability and there appears to be no particular cause for either symptoms improving or getting worse, with the exception that any kind of simple physical activity produces a generalised deterioration and fatigue, and rest seems to improve things. It is during this phase that patients feel at their most unwell and frequently are unable to specify what is wrong, simply saying 'I feel so ill'.

As time progresses the illness begins to mature and settle. There is more stability in the rate of change of symptoms which begin to diminish in severity and the exacerbations become much more predictable. Patients find themselves able to identify a frequently large number of complaints and problems in individual symptoms and that increasing physical and/or mental activity make the symptoms worse, seemingly in direct proportion to the amount of exertion or activity. Generally all of the symptoms are improved by both mental and physical rest and the patient learns by experience, like one of Pavlov's dogs, to avoid activities in both of these areas that worsen their symptoms and they tend to rest to improve them. This point of the clinical course might take you to one year from where the symptoms diminish and recovery continues. On the surface it would appear that the clinical course of AOPVFS is a naturally fluctuating one, there appears to be periods of worsening, mixed by improvement, setbacks, and cycles. Patients notice that not only do they suffer for their activities immediately, but that their recovery periods are extended frequently into several days or even a week if the activity had been particularly strenuous. The more vigorous the activity, the longer the period of punishment and the longer the period of recovery, during which, if any further activity is undertaken, either mental or physical, an apparent accumulative effect is noticed. The fatigue appears to pile up so that an exponential deterioration pattern is observed, leading to periods of illness that can be so bad that the patient appears to be 'pole-axed'. Recovery from these severe episodes can be quite extended and if the patient continues to push themselves to exhaustion, not only is the recovery from each of these episodes slower and longer but the whole illness can be extended in time and the degree of eventual 'illness' (termed 'morbidity') can be increased.

At this stage, persistent mishandling of the disease can lead to permanent ill health and perpetual morbidity. Usually, despite these generalised fluctuations the clinical progress demonstrates, albeit slowly, a tendency towards recovery. The periods of getting worse diminish in length and severity and the condition improves. As the severity of symptoms decline the level of activity is increased and as seen in Fig. 16 eventual recovery to point 'D' is almost complete.

Apart from mental and physical activity there are many other factors that influence the progress of recovery and interfere with return to full health. More usually however, the sufferer makes a fairly rapid recovery from these episodes, returning to previous levels of functioning. The most marked of these events being intercurrent infections. Here another 'cold' or 'flu-like' illness for which the symptoms are similar if not identical to those already being suffered produces a generalised exacerbation to a level that may enforce total rest. This tends to be short lived; possibly two, three or four weeks sees a return to previous levels. Recovery is expected to be far more rapid than the exacerbations seen in the 'over exercised' variety. However, any exacerbation leads to a further extension of the length of illness. Usually less deleterious effects are seen after general anaesthesia and operative procedures, trauma, broken limbs, road traffic accidents, etc. Vaccinations, especially with tetanus, typhoid and cholera have been observed to cause exacerbations for which recovery can be extremely slow and morbidity levels very high. Such vaccinations should therefore be avoided unless it is medically essential.

Quite marked increase in symptoms without actual exacerbations of the disorder are seen after a variety of things. Alcoholic beverages have a pronounced effect, making the general malaise and 'flu' like symptoms worse in some 70 per cent of patients with AOPVFS and many find themselves avoiding alcohol to the point of abstinence. Food sensitivity and intolerance can produce many of the symptoms, mainly those associated with irritable bowel syndrome, headache and painful joints. Many patients express other chemical intolerances (e.g. petrol fumes, gas, artificial preservatives, colourings and many others. The effects of these substances are discussed elsewhere but avoidance is probably the best form of treatment). These various intolerances have led to some of the most popular alternative forms of therapy in Post Viral Syndrome and M.E. – the exclusion diet and 'allergy' treatments. Whilst they can be helpful, one should be ever mindful that restrictive diets can be potentially hazardous and should always be pursued with medical advice.

The prognosis and outcome of AOPVFS

AOPVFS has a very large variety of levels of illness and morbidity. Figure 17 has the same vertical and horizontal axes as Figure 16 and represents the computerised average of some 1,500 personal graphs, all of which would be similar in type to that of the clinical course of typically unmanaged AOPVFS. The graphs in Figure 17 are a reflection of functional scores taken at illness intervals of six months from six months through to four years plus. The diagram starts at point 'A', an event that I would expect to happen to virtually everybody in Great Britain who suffers from 'flu'. It is that day on which anyone might develop an acute viral 'flu'-like infection and end up in bed. The vast majority would improve to full recovery and normal health from this infection in a period of approximately one week, represented by point 1 on the horizontal axis. Point 2 represents those that may recover over a more extended period of six to eight weeks. This would occur in a small proportion of the normal population, but whilst being unusual, would not be considered to be abnormal. If recovery has not occurred by six months as represented by the vertical dotted line, then the illness would meet the criteria for the diagnosis of AOPVFS (providing of course that other possible disorders have been excluded).

This failure to recover occurs in only a tiny fraction of the population suffering from an acute viral type infection. There are no epidemiological studies published on AOPVFS so far, and I was keen to get some idea about how many people in Great Britain might reach at least point 3 on the recovery scale so I decided to mail interested G.P.s, doctors who I knew were

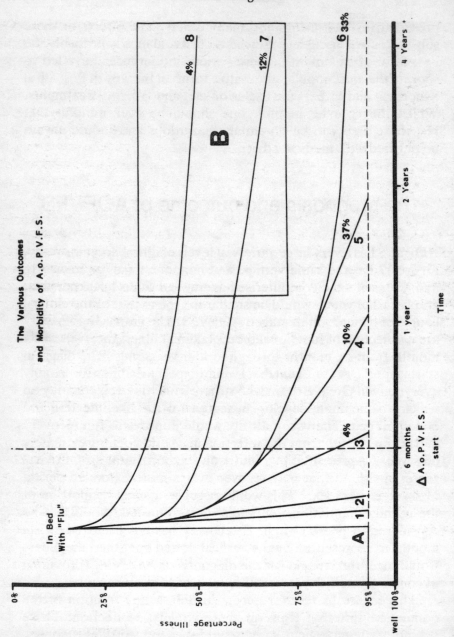

Fig 17. The various outcomes and morbidity of AOPVFS

prepared to make diagnosis of a Post Viral Syndrome, and ask them how many patients they thought they had, or had seen of one kind or another using whatever criteria they felt indicated that diagnosis. The reply was quite surprising; it suggested that the average practitioner saw two per year that had been ill for approximately one year or more.

Doing some rough back calculations about the number of patients that are registered with G.P.s and the number of G.P.s in Great Britain, gave the figure that the incidence of AOPVFS was one per thousand per head of the population of Great Britain who had an illness of at least one year. This would suggest that there are a great many more that are ill for less than one year and have recovered. It would be interesting to see how many there would be who were ill for say just six months and made an uneventful recovery. I suspect many more than the figure given above. However, the calculation would give a conservative nationwide total of 100,000 cases at any one time. Some other interesting facts come forth from Figure 17: it shows that about half of the disorder will recover spontaneously and completely within a period of approximately two years of onset i.e. by points 3, 4 and 5. By five years a further 33 per cent will have significantly improved but will remain at a low level of residual morbidity and I am quite sure that they never fully recover, and that they express the feeling that since the virus infection they have never been the same again, that they fatigue a little bit more than others, that they cannot pursue vigorous sporting activities or have too many late nights. Even if the illness has lasted five years there is always still a generalised tendency to improve; if they get worse, other possibilities other than a simple exacerbation of their AOPVFS should be considered.

There is however, a small but significant number, 16 per cent in whom higher levels of morbidity are seen and some 8 per cent have losses of 50 per cent of their function or more.

It is my opinion that medical mismanagement frequently contributes or even causes such permanent ill health. It is certainly responsible for a significant degree of morbidity. As an example, I have seen a number of patients, who after having been to see their General Practitioner or Consultant and having received a thorough clinical examination and appropriate investigations, are told that not only are the tests negative but there is simply nothing wrong with them and that they are psychologically disturbed, variously attributing the symptoms to hysterical conversion, depression, anxiety, or other neurotic illness. There is an unfortunate mistaken logic inherent in such an approach and I have discussed this elsewhere in this book. The patient that is faced with such an opinion tends to lie in box 'B' of Fig. 17. There are one or two interesting statistical facts that apply here: they tend to be rather older than average, they have a poor relationship with their spouse and family and they also tend to have difficulties with their doctors. It is not infrequent to find that the family has had a lot of discussion with the medical profession and views are expressed that frequently suggest that the ill member is simply 'putting it on'. By the time this situation has lasted a couple of years or so, such patients certainly do tend to have an increased percentage of psychiatric symptoms and problems. If you are told that you are psychologically disturbed often enough it may be that you become so. Skeletal muscle biopsies done in this group tend to show type 1 fibre atrophy, unfit skeletal muscle, reduction in mitochondrial levels, decreased muscle bulk and many of the changes that I have suggested are found in chronic disuse. Some have even shown fibrosis in the muscle, a totally irreversible disorder. One can see how they have developed this unfortunate self-fulfilling prophecy. I believe that they probably did not have any of these physical problems or psychiatric illness at the beginning of the disorder when they ended up in bed with flu, but as time goes by with entrenched attitudes both from the medical profession, and also let us remember from the patient, polarisation occurs, behavioural problems develop and the consequences of long standing ill health start. The numbers of patients that I have seen at points 3 and 4, are really very low, 4 per cent and 10 per cent respectively. It is not that there are so few patients but that the majority recover and are simply not referred and that patients tend to have to be ill for at least nine months to a year before referral starts. The larger proportion, 37 per cent at point 5 and 33 per cent at point 6 represents the majority of referral and also non recovery. I also believe that the numbers reflected in box 'B' of Fig. 17 are artificially low; this is because I have an influence on the referral. I have over the last three or four years started to refuse to see patients who have been ill for long periods of time, because

I have learned from experience that I cannot assist somebody who has been ill for five years or more and that if they do not have an acute viral type start to their disorder I am just not in a position to tell them what is going on; so rather than produce upset, anger and disappointment in the patient and a feeling of frustration in myself, I have turned them down.

I am seeing more cases at points 3 and 4 as interest in medicine continues to grow and a recognition of the disorder is taken up earlier. These patients are in groups that tend to recover and get good medical support and good advice. They are younger, in the age range of 16 to 40, with a peak at 32 years of age. They are in the main female (80 per cent), with good family support and even more importantly an interested and involved General Practitioner. They are the patients that have been told by their G.P. that they have some kind of Post Viral Syndrome and that even though their illness is not specifically managed, they are not given extremes of advice. They are encouraged to believe that they will get well within the 'near future'. Whilst this may of course be true, it is often found that these estimates for recovery times are a little optimistic. It appears that incorrect management at this stage is probably the reason that they do not recover within the expected six months or one year. If they do recover within that time then of course all is well.

However, if the anticipated recovery is not forthcoming the support from the family doctor wavers and questions begin, doubts begin to creep in and the accuracy of the diagnosis is questioned. Relatives, colleagues and doctors comment 'Isn't it about time you were better? Viruses can't last this long'. Everybody, including the patient, starts to wonder whether the illness is not due to something else and often the possibility is suggested that the illness was not viral but a psychiatric one after all. If this situation occurs such patients may experience a poor prognosis as those in box 'B' of Fig. 17. In my experience it is likely that those who end up with severe unremitting morbidity do so because of the medical non-management in the past. The severe psychiatric symptomatology and evidence of muscle disuse atrophy have both been acquired during the course of the illness and both were not present at the onset. The whole process has become a self-fulfilling prophecy by the doctors concerned. The condition of these patients can become apparently irrecoverable and this is certainly the case in a disease process of five or more years standing. In order to avoid this unfortunate situation in the future the patient's condition must be accurately identified much earlier in the course of their illness. Doctor and relatives need to communicate their understanding of the nature of the illness to the patient so that the patient knows they understand that he or she is 'ill' and that he or she is not then constantly having to prove that the illness is 'real'. Acceptance and appropriate management of the psychological symptoms is vital but this is not at all the same thing as telling the patient that the whole illness is psychiatrically based. The patient who is experiencing recurrent painful lymph glands, sore throats, severe muscle pain etc. will believe that the doctor is wrong, that they are missing something, possibly something serious and the patient will cease to have faith in the doctor's judgement and then polarise their own attitudes towards medicine and intransigence develops.

10
MANAGEMENT OF AOPVFS IN ADULTS AND HOW TO GET BETTER

The explanation

The most important aspect in the management is to be certain of the diagnosis, as the only therapeutic approach that *provably works* is that of correct disease management. This is a lengthy process and there is unfortunately no short cut. It requires a great deal of time and effort on behalf of not only the patient but also the physician and before going into the specific details of what to do a consultation should involve a detailed explanation not only to the patient but also their spouse, relatives, etc. about what is known of AOPVFS, and the fact that they have a recoverable process and that they are, in all probability, not going to be left permanently handicapped. They need encouragement and a discussion of problems that may go well beyond their immediate illness; it is important to understand the patient's life style, career, dependents, schooling etc. Most important of all is to get across to the patient that despite the fact that the illness may be a long one, a very positive approach is needed.

Identification of the exacerbating factors

Patients should be asked to keep a daily diary over the first few weeks into their management programme. This should not become too detailed or one can develop an introspective attitude, but a record of some kind can assist the patient to identify factors that influence their disease and then they see how long they suffer for doing some excessive activity. I usually suggest that they keep a daily temperature chart, preferably using one of the new electronic thermometers. This helps differentiate the symptoms of new virus infections from the reactivated ones, also to record the way that they feel in general terms and giving themselves a score out of 100 very much along the lines of the graph in Figure 2. I also ask them to keep a record of their degree of activity out of a top score of 10 and the minimal score of zero. You will then find patients can relate their degree of well-being to the degree of activity and they will be quickly rewarded by the identification of factors which influence their condition. At the following consultation which should be approximately 4–6 weeks later, their symptoms can be related to their activity graphically and the patient can be assisted in identifying obvious exacerbating features and ameliorating factors. This process will help the patient understand that *they are in control* of their own disease process and will see that a positive approach is an essential aid to recovery.

How much activity?

Good management is about getting patients better and this is dependent upon using the information in the subjective daily diary. Careful advice can then be given about how much activity should be undertaken, both from a physical and a mental point of view, in order to prevent increasing symptomatology and facilitate full recovery. How much activity initially advised depends upon the level of illness of the patient. Clearly more general activity can be suggested in those who are less afflicted and therefore a detailed statement is required about what activity is currently being undertaken and managed to date, without making the patient's symptoms worse. It is usually found that by the time the patient comes to referral that they have got some idea about the things that are making them worse and better and their illness tends to be on a plateau, neither getting worse nor better. Some on the other hand are clearly underdoing the activity and whilst their symptoms appear to be less they are not actually getting better, certainly not in functional terms. Lastly, and most commonly, the patients have been trying to push themselves because of advice they have given themselves or taken from elsewhere and their symptoms are fluctuating badly and the illness is getting worse, their activities are diminishing and the disease appears to be on a downward slide. Here the first thing to undertake is to stabilise the condition so that symptoms improve, allowing the disease process to settle. In order to understand the rationale of pacing 'power output' to achieve stabilisation in a modified activity programme, one needs to look at the way in which recovery is altered after physical or mental activity that occurs in patients suffering from AOPVFS.

By comparing 'power output' and the recovery times in normal individuals and patients suffering from AOPVFS, one can see a healthy but untrained individual would not expect to suffer for more than a day. After a one mile jog, they would, however, expect to have mild muscle aches and pains and fatigue which would completely recover within twenty-four hours.

In comparison a patient suffering mildly from AOPVFS, who might be capable of a one mile jog, finds that she suffers from excessive fatigue and increased symptoms. The recovery from this is seen to be extended into several days.

Fig. 18 shows that by constantly trying to produce a maximum power output the patient with AOPVFS can cause a relapse or at least a severe exacerbation of symptoms. As the example, Fig. 18, graph A represents the maximum work output and recovery in a normal individual. Graph B is that of a person suffering from AOPVFS in which the recovery time is extended. If as suggested by C further power is expended when there has not been an adequate recovery from the activity undertaken in B, then the recovery time of C is seen to be longer and slower and also the power output achieved is lessened, they simply can't do as much. The same applies to graph D where the power output is further reduced. The recovery is again further diminished and it appears that with a relatively minor power output to point E is followed by the patient experiencing an exacerbation and a feeling of being 'pole-axed' or 'wiped out'. Any further power production appears impossible and results in a return to total rest and even bed from which the recovery process can be very slow, taking several days. As they improve their 'power output' again begins to rise and as recovery is sustained the 'power output' can often be pushed too far yet again, causing another relapse. The features of Fig. 18 are seen time and time again when talking to patients who are not managing their disease process well. Where one elicits stories of 'ups and downs', good days, bad days, good weeks, bad weeks which are all too common. When this 'knock on' effect of fatigue after effort is not understood patients believe that the illness fluctuates in a haphazard fashion and that there appears to be no rhyme or reason for the way that they feel. This is not the case and the disorder *IS NOT* a naturally fluctuating one, it is indeed highly predictable.

Similar graphs to Fig. 18 can be produced using a vertical axis of mental activity or 'stress and strain' which produces increased fatigue both mentally and physically and with enough mental stress and strain exacerbations can be seen to be produced in exactly the same fashion as that produced by the power output. There is a very close relationship between over production of power and excessive mental stress and strain. They appear to be frequently indivisible and mutually summatory. By understanding how this power output or mental stress and strain can generate relapses one can develop a disease management programme to aid initially the stabilisation of the illness and then its subsequent improvement.

If you sit and think about this problem for just a few moments, the amount of physical activity or mental output that is optimum for the condition becomes very obvious. Too little in the way of activity is undesirable, non-progressive, and bad for you (see later). Too much activity produces an exacerbation. The answer *must* lie somewhere in between.

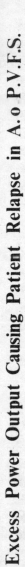
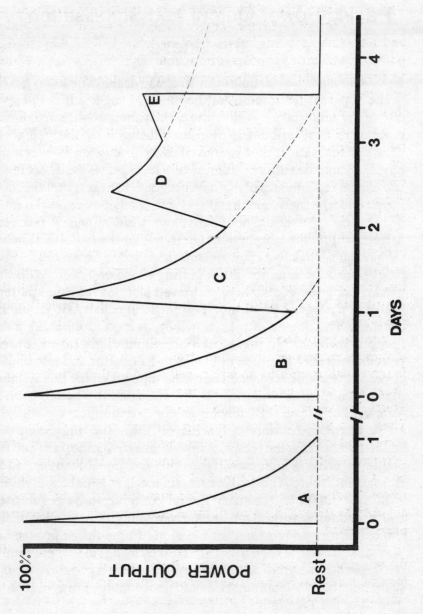

Fig. 18 Excess power output causing patient relapse in AOPVFS

Pacing Power Output and Stabilisation of the Illness

By pacing one's power output in a regular fashion one can get rid of the apparent fluctuations of the illness. I suggest that the level of activity undertaken is much less than the patient's maximum capability. That amount is of course dictated by the degree of illness of the patient and is arrived at by discussion between the physician and the sufferer. It must be a level that is easily achieved and can be repeated regularly day after day. I suggest that the level is well underpitched; and that this level of daily power output must be the same, and should not fluctuate very much then. A recovery pattern will then be observed. There will of course be a residual fatigue but each daily activity is superimposed upon a fixed level of recovery, so the situation is not getting worse or better. With this 'pacing' a period of stability is achieved and this repeated pattern becomes a programme of modified physical activity. It should be constant. The degree of mental activity is monitored in a similar fashion. Using such a regularised programme, improvement will be seen to occur. The patient begins to feel better and less unwell as the fluctuations are ironed out. The time taken for this stability to start is individual and variable, but in someone who has been ill for a year or so will probably be one or two months.

As this period of stability is achieved, the improving patient will begin to notice that the recovery time after activity shortens and the degree of recovery increases. It then becomes possible to suggest an increase in activity. The degree of increment is negotiable but should *always* be small. The activity should continue to be regularised and paced for several days, thus maintaining the stability of the clinical picture and again after a period of time the improvement in symptoms will be seen to occur. Thus by using small incremental steps, the disease gradually remits and recovery is progressive. It is suggested that the increments should not be made more frequently than once per fortnight.

Such a gradual recovery programme is essential, as is the advice that too much rest is as bad if not worse than too much activity. Prolonged periods of rest are to be avoided wherever possible as they lead to a perpetuation of the very symptoms being complained of.

Each patient requires an individual programme of *daily* activity and splitting the day up into smaller periods of rest and activity both mental and physical is advocated especially in the earlier acute phases of the disease where the symptoms are more fluid and mobile. The ratio of mental to physical activity depends not only upon the severity of the symptoms but the relative preponderance of mental/physical which can be markedly different from one patient to another. It is better to divide activities into small periods throughout the day, as an example, two quarter hour walks at either end of the day are more rewarding and less fatiguing than one half hour walk. The same kind of rationale should be applied to mental study which should be based upon the assessment of the degree of concentration or memory seen in the patient's capacity for reading a book or a newspaper.

This then becomes a basic programme for mental and physical activity and should be repeated to the same level every day for approximately two weeks or so. There should be *no* uncontrolled outbursts of strenuous activity and the regime is rigorous, and of necessity, rather monotonous. After this introductory programme the clinical response is reassessed and it will be found that the marked fluctuations in the illness will have disappeared or at least lessened because of the control of the pattern of activity which secures the 'punishment time-lag effect'. The patient should be found to be at least as well, if not better, than they were before. If the patient's symptoms are worse and the fatigue more pronounced then the programme of activity may need to be cut back. If their condition remains unchanged the programme is continued for another similar period of time, at the same level of activity. The usual course, however, is to find the patient improved and feeling better and thus it can be suggested that both the mental and physical activity should be increased by a very small amount at the expense of the rest periods. It is, however, most important that stabilisation of the clinical picture is achieved. This is the key stone to improving recovery. After which time the activity is increased by small amounts in a slow, incremental fashion. This part of the rehabilitation is a good time to regularise the times of getting up in the morning and going to bed at night. This is particularly important for the sufferer in employment or attending school who should try and return to a normal waking

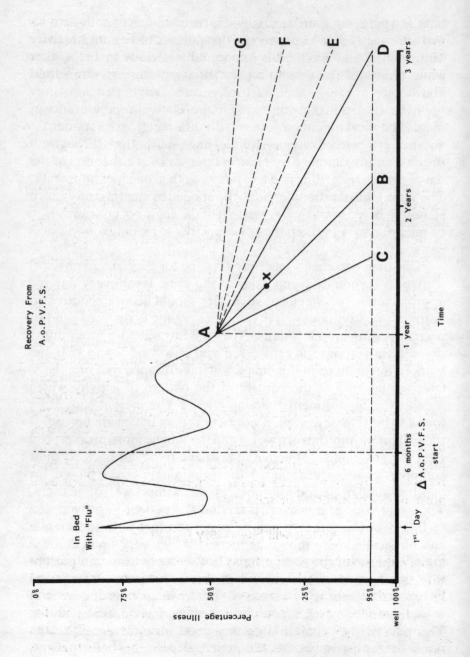

Fig. 19 Recovery from AOPVFS

time in preparing for the day when they are ready to return to work or education. By adopting this graduated activity programme. The sufferer prevents the likelihood of deleterious exacerbations which lead so frequently to a substantial extension of the whole illness.

Returning to Work

The same graduated approach should be used when returning to work, school or college. It will be necessary to discuss this transitional phase with the work's doctor, occupational physician or welfare officer as appropriate. A gradual return starting with simply one or two half days per week is advised, and maintaining that level for a month, before building up slowly to full-time. This should always be done at a rate of increase of one or two half days at a time and not more frequent than at monthly intervals, so it can be a considerable time before full-time work is resumed.

Where the illness is unfortunately a long one, patients can frequently find themselves being pressured into returning to work or school far too soon by threats of job loss, retirement on medical grounds etc. These pressures in themselves trigger anxiety, depression and mental stress and actively exacerbate the disease process and its recovery. Alleviation of these pressures by suitable and appropriate discussions wherever possible is very important, so that everybody has a full understanding of how recovery is likely to occur and a progress towards return to a normal life, occupation or schooling.

When will Recovery Occur?

Fig. 19 shows the graph of a typical recovery pattern of a patient suffering from AOPVFS in whom fluctuations are seen caused by exacerbations and remissions in the unmanaged case and who themselves might present for advice after being ill for approximately one year, suggested here at point A. The axes are the same as for Fig. 16, the patient despite these fluctuations has made an improvement of some 25% in functional terms. Using the management programme suggested earlier one might expect

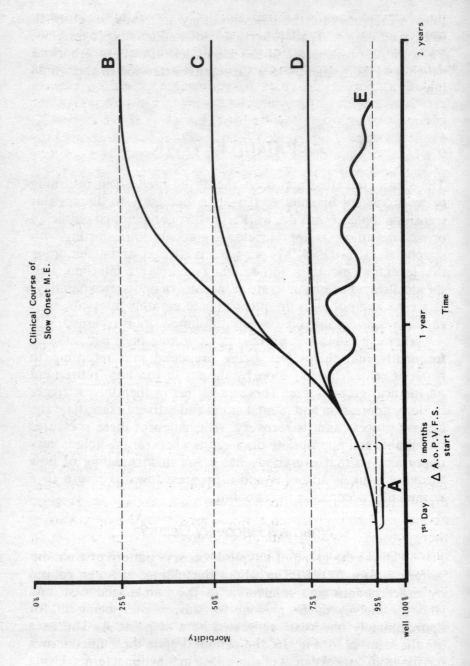

Fig. 20 Clinical course of slow onset M.E.

improvement along the solid lines of B, C or D making the recovery time two years two months, one year seven months, or three years respectively. At the initiation of a management programme at point A the outcome is uncertain except to say that eventually the patient is likely to improve. If the patient is reviewed at two and four months into the management programme they might return indicating a rate of improvement which if plotted on the graph would be at point X. From this point it is possible to extrapolate in the direction of the 'Fit Line' striking it at point B, giving a forecasted recovery date of just over two years. If, however, the patient returns after a management programme instigation and suggests a greater rate of improvement then the forecast may be improved to point C. Equally a slower improvement may be unfortunately indicated and recovery delayed to point D. As discussed earlier, Fig. 17, once the second year of illness has been reached, the recovery appears not to be linear and the impetus is lost and tends to tail off leaving some degree of eventual morbidity, here suggested variably by the hatched lines reaching points E, F and G.

From my observations, I am sceptical that if the illness has extended beyond two and a half years that recovery can ever be complete although there is always a tendency to improve long term. Most patients with an illness of less than two years do reach a level of almost full recovery but many do appear to have minor residual complaints suggesting that their fitness and strength has never been quite the same as prior to the illness.

The capability of being able to tell a patient that they will recover is of course of great importance and I have found that the rate of recovery in AOPVFS is quite predictable. No other disease process appears to have the same degree of certainty about the slow progression towards recovery. Having said this, there are unfortunately patients who do not recover and remain ill for reasons that are not immediately apparent. Whatever the causes for this protracted illness are, it becomes more certain that the factor to getting patients well and fully recovered is to be able to intercept the illness and to instigate a management programme at the earliest possible time. Generally if the illness can be detected and intercepted before one year, then recovery is virtually guaranteed.

The Management of Slow Onset M.E.

By introducing the tight disease diagnostic criteria in definition of AOPVFS there are necessarily a large number of fatigued patients excluded from that diagnosis. There can be no possible disease definition that encompasses all fatigue syndromes and subsets found within the M.E. umbrella. However, in my earlier studies I used to see a lot of patients who had similar symptoms to those of AOPVFS but not the initiating 'viral type' story. The history was lacking a particular start, they tended on the whole to have an insidious onset and their problems tended to become gradually worse, more persistent and very tenacious.

If one applies similar restraints in the diagnosis as seen in the definition of AOPVFS by excluding patients who have other significant problems or previous histories of serious illness, then one might be left with a group of patients with an unexplained fatigue syndrome that could not be justifiably said to be purely psychiatrically based and for whom modern organic medicine has no convincing answer. In this situation such a disorder might be referred to as slow onset M.E. Figure 20 shows the clinical course of slow onset M.E. at four different morbidity levels. It again uses the same axes for Fig. 16 and it suggests that patients who were previously fit and well until a time incorporated in the bracket 'A' when their disease process appears to begin. Because when it starts there is often no obvious predisposing factor or event. Their illness continues to become more severe and there appears to be a whole variety of morbidity. As suggested here by the severe case of B through to the lesser illness of D.

There are several features of this disorder that are different from AOPVFS, there are fewer cases that spontaneously get better. The majority appear to plateau out and their clinical condition has much less in the way of fluctuation of symptoms. However, increased mental and physical activity, stress and strain make their symptoms generally worse, as does rest make them better. The fluctuations are much less marked and they show an increased tendency to chronicity and if anything tend to deteriorate. It is also of interest to note that the sex ratio in this group is roughly 50 per cent male to female. They tend to be older and the psychiatric symptoms are less florid in the early stages of M.E. than in the acute stages of AOPVFS, but depression is far more frequent.

I have always had a great deal of trouble in managing this large fatigue subset and it appears that their problems are more intransigent. Antidepressants are less effective, modified activity programmes and behavioural therapy do not help as much in this group. They appear to have a very poor prognosis. I am sure that there are many disease possibilities here and the management of that disease necessarily depends upon the identification of the underlying process and the management is far more open to discussion.

There is however, a small sub-group of the slow onset M.E. that I have suggested improve. The symptoms and the clinical picture become more like that of AOPVFS, it is more fluctuating in symptomatology and tends to respond more to antidepressants and modified activity programmes. It is clear that here also the best response is seen in the disease that is managed in the earlier stages and it is to all intents and purposes clinically the same as AOPVFS (see — group E in Fig. 20) but without the story so suggestive of the acute viral start.

Too much rest is bad for you

There is no doubt that too much rest is bad for you, even if you are well and especially when we talk about M.E. or Post Viral Syndrome. As we get older, our natural drive and instincts to 'keep on going' tend to diminish. When one reaches that magical middle age, indolence seems to swell up in most of us, and with our diminishing activities there is no commensurate drop off in appetite and we tend to spread. All normal enough, I am afraid, and these changes are better adjusted to by some people and less by others. We all have enormously variable levels of activity, there are those that are always on the go and a few sloths, but altogether that pattern is simply a reflection of normal individuals.

These various changes that begin to occur normally in early middle life are also at the time that most frequently sees M.E. and AOPVFS develop.

If I take perfectly normal, middle-aged individuals, and put them to bed for three days the symptoms that they will complain of when getting out of bed are fatigue, muscle aches and pains and weakness. Put them to bed for one or two weeks then boredom and depression are added to the list and the other symptoms are simply worse. They are also the very symptoms of M.E. They are the symptoms that cause the sufferer to stop and to take rest, either self imposed, or advised. If they are the symptoms that make you go to bed and the symptoms that you develop once you are there, where does one begin and the other one stop?

To understand this a little bit more one has to look at the biochemical and metabolic changes that occur in muscle during rest.

Muscle is by far the largest bulk of tissue in the body and if it does not work properly you are going to get an awful lot of complaints from it. Muscles are made up of fibres. They contain contractile protein that is provided with energy supplied by mitochondria. Each fibre is filled with millions of minute egg-shaped structures called mitochondria which contain a whole series of enzymes designed to break nutrients down into energy and waste products. They are literally little power houses.

A normal individual who decides upon a training programme to get fit in any method that you care to choose, will slowly increase their total muscle bulk. They do not actually increase the number of muscle fibres, but the fibres increase in mass, they get bigger in the cross sectional area, with an increase in the contracting protein and a vast increase in the numbers of mitochondria. The availability then of energy to the contractile system is substantially increased. Training and getting fit is a slow process, you have to really work at it. Getting unfit, on the other hand, is rapid and is much easier. I am quite sure that the majority of you, possibly by first hand experience, have seen the effects of sticking a large piece of plaster on to a broken bone or a bad sprain, keep that on for two, three or four weeks, and then take the plaster off and lo and behold the veritable 'withered arm'. It is amazing, the flesh just simply disappears, it seems to melt away and it did not take long. The same happens if you go to bed or rest too much, the muscles initially become generally unfit and then the bulk begins to disappear. If you look at them under the microscope, the cross sectional area of the fibre is decreased, the contractile material is diminished and the numbers of mitochondria that produce power for the whole system also reduce. This last process takes only a few days, the actual muscle proteins and muscle bulk might take some weeks to become noticeably diminished. To reverse this situation frequently takes months if not a year and one has to exercise them to quite a high level to recover. Witness the agonies that one goes through trying to get a broken limb mobilised again to its original strength. One cannot take that sort of rehabilitation with Post Viral Syndrome and M.E. but certainly if you rest too much I hope that you can see that one is going to get biochemical and structural changes occurring that can be very difficult to reverse and a very long time in coming.

I have even seen the advice that says, 'stop before you get tired'. I hope that you will see how unreasonable that advice must be. If I, as a relatively busy, healthy individual, stopped before I got tired, I would finish work at 5 p.m. This slothful behaviour would only increase my tiredness and by the end of the second week I would be feeling tired at 4 p.m, or 3 p.m. and by the end of a month I think that I would be in bed. Stay three days in bed and you have the symptoms of M.E. So adopting that advice would find you permanently, irrevocably bed bound and you have just obtained a self-fulfilling prophecy. What are the consequences of longer periods of rest, of say one month or more? That degree of immobility must automatically mean that the patient is at least housebound, either lying in bed or sitting in a chair all the time. There is no stimulation, one reverts to television, radio, reading, hobbies, computer games and the like. One becomes introspective, thoughtful and more aware of bodily symptoms, aches and pains. Social withdrawal leads to depression after an initial period of being fed up and low, and there is no doubt that most lose their friends and families find it difficult and they become frustrated and intolerant. Sleep patterns change, eating patterns change, too much or too little seems to be fairly common with the commensurate problems then of increasing weight or anorexia. Hormonal fluctuations that are normal in the healthy individual begin to change and there is a natural fluctuation in the amount of steroids produced by the adrenal glands. These are needed for all sorts of fluctuating bodily functions that occur in the day and these fluctuations are called 'diurnal variation' and this tends to stop when you are bed bound. Normal, naturally fluctuating daily temperature changes also stop. The metabolism alters, bones begin to thin, bowels begin to dysfunction, usually with constipation and the whole life force of the body begins to slide.

These changes are not peculiar to M.E. or AOPVFS. They are common to every chronic severely dehabilitating disease, but unlike AOPVFS and M.E. most other diseases are treated by physiotherapy and by increased encouragement and activity. Also unlike the majority of other chronic disease processes which are slow in their progress, AOPVFS by definition is a sudden, frequently pole-axing disorder that occurs in a fit and healthy person. From being physically fit and active one day, the sufferer can be devastated the next. So the sudden imposition of enforced diminished activity is that much more acute than the chronic type of disease.

I am of course aware that there are going to be periods when some patients are confined to bed or to resting in a chair, especially in the earlier times of their disease. I hope that I am making just some of you aware of the changes that occur in the rested patient and that when rest has occurred for several weeks or months that both the physical and mental changes that occur can be profound. Patients need long term rehabilitation programmes and that resting in itself when unchecked and unmonitored is potentially a malignant process.

11
WHY ME?

It is not possible to provide a definite answer to the question as to who is likely to be affected by M.E. until we know precisely what the disease is, and whether there is just one cause or a multiple aetiology. We need a qualified epidemiologist to do an extensive study of M.E. to provide the solution. The following paragraphs, then, are nothing more than reasonable suggestions – and I do mean reasonable; there are many other possibilities put forward which I personally feel are unlikely.

Let us have a look at the group of people suffering from AOPVFS. I must straightaway point out that I have not encountered any epidemics; the patients that I have seen are sporadic cases. They come from all over the country, so the first question is:

Geographical location: Do they come from any particular place? Well, at the moment, the answer to that must be no. The greatest number of people I see are from the home countries, but that is not surprising, because that is where the greatest population is. After that there seems to be a very homogenous spread throughout the whole of Great Britain.

On the international scale, M.E. is a phenomenon which is widespread throughout the world, cases in the United States, Canada, New Zealand and Australia being the most commonly reported. Here, however, they seem to be of the epidemic variety, where a particular city suffers an outbreak.

As to other parts of Europe, I am not sure whether the diagnosis of AOPVFS is yet being made. The same point must apply to Africa, where they have much more serious diseases, such as AIDS, typhoid and cholera to contend with, apart from much more in the way of enterovirus infection and, indeed, an extra Coxsackie B thrown in for good measure.

Race or religion: There does not appear to be any colour or creed influence that I can see at the present, although my initial impression is that it is a Caucasian disorder. Out of a thousand patients I have seen only two Indians, both of whom had spent most of their life in England.

Diets or chemical exposure: As you can see from the questionnaire, we asked a lot of questions about chemical exposures, stresses, a predisposing candidiasis problem, antibiotics, food insensitivity etc. Unfortunately the results at the moment are not suitable for analysis but two points came over quite clearly; the first was that the vast majority had stopped drinking alcohol (see pp. 228–29), the second that many had expressed some food intolerance (see pp. 224–5). There did not appear to be any significant predisposing atopy or allergy problems in patients with AOPVFS as opposed to the general population. There were no people on peculiar diets prior to their disease starting.

With regard to antibiotics, those who had sore throats at the beginning of the disorder – 6 per cent – received antibiotics at the time. Those who complained of intermittent recurrent sore throats, a much larger number, were given antibiotics later in their clinical course. None of the people whom I looked at prior to the study and subsequent to it had any significant exposure to antibiotics prior to the onset of their disorder. I do not believe that antibiotic therapy, or mistherapy, contributes to the instigation of AOPVFS.

Chemical exposure showed a total zero, none of the patients recalling any incidence of this.

Subsequent to the trial, I did see one lady who was convinced that she became ill after being in quite close contact with a hoya plant!

Stress: The majority of people claimed that they had been experiencing work, relationship, or marital problems for some three to six months prior to their virus.

Sex: A remarkable phenomenon is that 85 per cent of those people suffering from AOPVFS are female. Why this should be is not yet established.

Age: I am unhappy about making the diagnosis of this disorder under the age of twelve. Indeed, I am getting more cautious about making it under the age of fifteen. I am certain that it occurs but the phenomenon gets much more confused with inter-family and parental reaction.

So, starting from about fifteen, the age of onset peaks at thirty-two, and becomes almost a rarity after forty. I am not yet sure why this should be so.

Socio-economic status: There has been a lot of media hype about 'yuppy flu' but I am quite convinced that the typical M.E. patient is a young middle-aged housewife. Ninety-five per cent of my patients are married and 85 per cent of those have children. The majority (62 per cent) were working prior to their disease onset, and their jobs were various. Undoubtedly there were some high pressured jobs, for example in advertising agencies and hospitals, but most patients classified themselves mainly as housewives with jobs. They had young children and were being at the same time mother, bread-winner and housekeeper, which is of course extremely hard work and very stressful.

There is no reason to suppose that the patients I have seen are not representative of the general population of M.E. sufferers. Consequently, what I have quoted here can be taken as a true reflection of the type of person most likely to suffer from M.E. and its sub-group AOPVFS.

Why do we get M.E.?

Abnormal immunological process

There is no doubt that stress plays an important part in the development of AOPVFS, and there is convincing immunological evidence to suggest that people under stress do not make an appropriate immune response. If people are placed under stress in laboratory experiments their T and B-cell function can be found to be abnormal and humoural agents (chemicals which are released during the immunological process) are also abnormal. So it is possible that under stressful conditions we do not produce the right amounts of antibody, or that the antibody produced is not effective, and here one must also consider predisposing psychological status.

People under stress are, in the broader sense of the word, often also depressed, and studies have been done to show that depressed people exposed to a virus infection take longer to recover, and have a temperature for a longer period of time, than people who are not stressed or depressed. Other studies actually show that people who are under stress or depressed, or both, actually get more virus infections than those who are not. So here one can see clear evidence of the relationship of the psyche with organic infective disease.

Genetic origin

At the point of conception we are endowed with the genetic material that allows our white cells to develop and to make an appropriate response to various antigens. Is there, therefore, a missing or an inadequate gene that means that the body cannot express the appropriate immunoglobulins or effect a normal immunological response? I really do not know the answer to this, but there are a few points that I would like to make that suggest that this is unlikely.

The first is that if there were a genetic abnormality, the clinical picture of the highest incidence of the disorder in females aged thirty-two would not be the commonest pattern; one would tend to see it more, I believe, in younger people, and also the older age group as they came across the virus to which they could not react.

The second point is that if there were a genetic inability to respond appropriately, I would not expect people to get better – their disease process would tend to continue, which is not the actual clinical picture that one observes.

Thirdly, in those outbreaks that occur in epidemic form, many people go down with the disorder and do not immediately recover.

It seems unlikely that there could be a genetic influence here; the evidence is more pointed towards the virulence of the virus at that time, rather than an abnormal genetically determined host response.

To confirm absolutely whether or not there is any genetic predisposition, however, one needs to look at tissue typing, and this we are doing.

Lack of rest

It may be that at the time of the initial virus infection that precipitates their AOPVFS the patient does not rest appropriately. Unfortunately we did not include a question on that in the study, but there is a lot of evidence that inadequate rest, as far as the enteroviruses are concerned, may be responsible for subsequent problems.

Inadequate rest does not appear to play an important part in the pathogenesis of disease in other viruses such as chickenpox or hepatitis. However, with regard to the enteroviruses, it was discovered that if a patient with polio was totally confined to bed for three to six months the outcome of the paralytic aftermath was less. The polio viruses are structurally identical to the other 72 enteroviruses and the method of infection is the same, so there may well be an argument that inadequate rest during the initial phase of the acute upper respiratory tract infection or flu-like illness caused by the enteroviruses leads to the subsequent development of M.E. and/or AOPVFS. On the whole, however, I believe that the development of AOPVFS has more to do with the virulence of the virus at the time of the initial infection.

Viral virulence

The enteroviruses do not change their shape or their antigenic structure, but each one of them is capable of being either very potent or relatively impotent.

Let us take a hypothetical case of a child with an enterovirus 'cold'. A throat swab taken in the very early days of the infection can be found to cause widespread cellular damage and death to cells on a culture plate. A sample can be taken from that culture plate and moved to another, where the same effect can be seen;

however, after this process is repeated several times, the amount of cellular damage and death that occurs on the culture plate diminishes – in other words, the virus becomes less pathogenic. The reason for this is that the virus develops defective interfering particles (DI particles). During the very first cell culture, all of the virus that was introduced was infective particles. Once they are introduced into a cell, the virus particles made inside that cell are sometimes genetically imperfect and contain shorter sequences of RNA genome. These virus particles, while still maintaining an effective cellular penetration to other cell mediums, tend to reproduce themselves and the resultant infective particle is not so virulent and does not kill so many cells. As the number of defective particles begin to rise, there is a competitive situation between the virulent virus and the defective virus. The higher the concentration of the defective virus, the lower the incidence of cell death in serial cell culture.

Let us take that observed laboratory fact to the clinical situation. Little Johnny, aged seven, comes home from school with a nasty enterovirus cold; Father is out at work each day but Mother stays at home to look after her ailing son. In the first few days of Johnny's illness he is extremely infectious, coughing his virulent virus from the back of his throat towards his mother, who picks up a highly pathogenic dose of enterovirus, succumbs to the same illness, and goes on to develop AOPVFS as a result. At some stage the pathogenesis of this virus changes and become less infective; Father develops a much less virulent infection a week later and makes a normal response, recovering easily. He may not even develop the full clinical disease, merely suffering a minor sneeze, so you can see how an explanation of an initial aggressive virus, which can be more passive as time goes by, could answer some of the developmental problems of AOPVFS.

Viral dose

Let us take our little Johnny analogy again. If he came home from school with his enterovirus, gave his father a peck on the cheek and a much more affectionate kiss to his mother, and then sneezed over a brother or so, they would all be subjected to variable amounts of virus – Father might get twenty viruses, Mother half a million, siblings a few hundred thousand. Even if the virus were at the same potency, it would not be unreasonable for Mother to go down with the worst infection because she had received a larger dose of virus. Consequently she may be the one who goes on to produce ΛOPVFS, while the others recover. In truth, the development and the severity of the illness probably depends upon combinations of viral dose, pathogenicity and the host response.

The Development of Persistence of Enterovirus Infection

In August of 1990, a paper was written and published in the Journal of General Virology (Reference 1) and it has taken the understanding for the development of persistent enterovirus infections, a very large step further forward. Len Archard was one of the authors, and I know him quite well, so I decided to go and discuss this paper with him to get a better understanding of precisely what is going on.

The work was done on muscle biopsies sent to him from Peter Behan in Glasgow and also taken locally at Charing Cross Hospital. The patients, described as suffering from Chronic Fatigue Syndrome, were complaining of excessive muscle fatigue ability following some kind of presumed virus infection and to all intents and purposes they fulfilled the diagnostic criteria of Chronic Fatigue Syndromes put forward by Holmes et al in 1988 (Reference 2).

The story of the development of persistent enterovirus infection would suggest that the majority of us suffer from these extremely common viruses in a subclinical way which means that the patient really would hardly know that they were ill. There would probably be either no symptoms at all or just the mildest, usually a simple cold or a gastro-intestinal upset. This type probably accounts for well over 80 per cent of all virus infections including the enteroviruses. They are self limiting probably because the viral dose is not adequate to sustain a 'roll on' effect. In the clinical type of infection, if you like the next stage up, one would expect an involvement of the nose and the back of the throat, a Laryngitis or Pharyngitis as they would be termed. This infection would have the symptoms of a runny nose, sore throat, a cough and a temperature. Here, the virus would be neutralised by the production of a surface antibody

IgA response, previously discussed elsewhere. This IgA response is not entirely specific for that virus but is certainly adequate in eliminating the majority. However, if the virus takes a deeper hold, it might travel further down to the gastro-intestinal system by-passing the stomach acid, (as they are acid resistant) where they develop a more extensive infection. The virus would infect and start reproducing itself in the lymphatic tissue which lines the intestines. This would be an intestinal or enteric infection and the virus at this stage becomes more invasive, passing through the lymphatic tissue and in the lymph fluid where it would percolate throughout the body. This stimulates a blood borne response by the body, termed a humoral response, goading the lymphocytes to make an IgM antibody response. There is also a generalised interferon production. You will recall that interferon is the substance that gives rise to the typical 'flu' like symptoms of a virus infection that we would all recognise. They are headache, fever, malaise, muscle aches and pains, and feeling non-specifically ill.

After a few days, somewhere between three and ten, one would typically see the immune system making a long term antibody response using the specific IgG production which would neutralise the virus. This leads to recovery which happens to virtually everybody. In the small percentage of people that go on to develop AOPVFS, it is suggested that the following happens. At the stage where the virus becomes blood borne, and stimulating a production of interferon, the virus penetrates various cells of the body. It depends upon the type of virus as to exactly which cells they invade, but in the case of the enteroviruses, they have a predilection to go to muscle and nervous tissue. As the virus enters the cell it leaves a mark on the surface and in doing so leaves the immune system capable of mounting an inflammatory response. T Lymphocytes are mobilised and as they recognise the cells that have this surface mark, they mature into killer cells opening up the infected cell and destroying the virus inside, killing the cell in the process. If you open up too many cells the patient is not going to survive. Of course there are a few people who do get overwhelming virus infections and succumb, but fortunately death is not a very common event in the majority of virus infections. So, hopefully in this particular instance, the number of cells that are infected are not too great, the viruses are hunted down and eliminated.

It is after penetration of the cell that an alteration in viral replication occurs and may provide us with the explanation of how AOPVFS develops. The enteroviruses are single stranded RNA viruses and during their multiplication, because they do not have a matching template as seen in the DNA viruses, which can rectify errors, the RNA strands read like a book, from one end to the other, and having no checking mechanism they are open to develop errors which they do at an alarming rate. Viruses that develop errors are imperfect and are in fact mutants. It has been found that RNA viruses should 'read', in other words, reproduce themselves in one direction. The normal way is supposed to be in a positive direction (say from left to right) but in the muscle samples produced from Glasgow it was found that the virus was frequently (50%) being read backwards and also that the virus proteins, VP1, VP2, VP3 and VP4 which are used to make up the viral capsule are no longer being produced. It is these virus proteins when expressed on the surface of the cell that stimulate an antigenic response from the T Lymphocytes. When these proteins are missing, and are not expressed, lymphocytes no longer have a target. The virus replication inside is hidden from our immune system by the cell membrane itself. This defective replication renders the virus useless as an infective agent, as it is not complete. Inside the cell they are just bits of virus, a series of RNA sequences. The body cannot eradicate them, so they simply sit there taking over the cell's function to make more RNA. The defective replication of RNA continues and is theoretically capable of doing so ad infinitum. These RNA sequences are broken down inside the cell by an enzyme called Ribonuclease and this happens quite quickly, every ten minutes or so, thus the virus, RNA has to multiply at less than ten minutes. This amount of activity inside the cell must cause some inefficiency and prevent normal performance of other functions. It is causing a tremendous waste of energy and will diminish the executive function of that particular cell, in the case of muscle it would reduce the cell's capability of producing powerful contractions. One could imagine that if this situation does carry on for ever and if enterovirus infection is the cause of AOPVFS or at least some cases of it, then the development of this type of persistent infection would easily answer the continuing symptoms and problems of muscle fatigue.

So how can this constant RNA replication stop, how can you get better from it? One possible explanation is the fact that there is a host response that has an effect upon these RNA mutations. It has been noticed that during these various experiments the genetic mutations that occur are not always the same. The breaks in the chain of RNA synthesis tend to be in the same place in one particular person's muscle, but not the same in another. This suggests that there must be some kind of host response that has an effect upon these breaks and that the person being infected appears to have some part to play in where these defects occur. It may be that this host response is genetically pre-determined, despite the fact that there are previous HLA typing studies which suggest that there is not any genetic predisposition to the development of AOPVFS or M.E. Probably the more important point in how one might get better is that the various mutations tend, if anything, to be slowly progressive. In other words as time goes by more mutations occur. At some point if the mutation does not include the production of various enzymes that are necessary in the RNA sequences, the whole thing is likely to suddenly grind to a halt, and they self destruct. This self limiting switch off one assumes can occur at any time within minutes of the initial infection or possibly many years later.

There are other situations in which a host genetic response appears to be a specific requirement to the development of a persistent enterovirus infection. This is seen in laboratory work that is done upon the development of various infections seen in animals. For instance if you are trying to produce an animal model to help you with the understanding of a virus infection of the heart called myocarditis then you not only need a very specific strain of Coxsackie B3 virus called 'Nancy' but you also need a special type of male mouse called 'Touson'. You have to put these two together before you will develop a particular virus type of reaction that provokes an infection in the heart muscle. Recent work being done at some of the heart transplant centres show that there may be a genetic predisposition required to the development of a particularly nasty enterovirus infection of the heart muscle in humans. Fortunately this is extremely rare. The virus continues to produce an infection in the heart muscle and develop a disorder called dilated cardiomyopathy. This condition leads to a very slowly dilating heart, the cure for which is usually transplant and initial studies look as though there is a particular type of genetic factor at work here. In other words, certain people of a certain genetic type are predisposed to getting this disorder after a particular enterovirus virus.

Persistent enterovirus infection is certainly not the cause of everybody's AOPVFS, indeed it is probably only a small percentage. This kind of enterovirus RNA mutations that are described are certainly not the answer to all the other findings of AOPVFS. For instance they cannot be responsible for the VP1 test. The VP1 test is the detection of virus protein 1, an antigen detected in the blood. As these RNA mutations inside the muscle cell are not expressing virus protein antigens on the surface of the cell, they cannot produce them, and therefore the fact that VP1 is positive in some people must be answered by the fact that these virus proteins are being made somewhere else and not in the muscle tissue. There must be a constant production of active infective virus to continually produce this VP1. Presumably this source of virus is an active reproduction that comes from somewhere else like the gut or the throat. Intermittent or even persistent sore throats are common in AOPVFS as is the apparent glandular enlargement or at least occurrence of tender glands, not only in the neck but also the armpits and the groin. It would not seem unreasonable that we should look for active whole infective virus replication in these areas.

These sites are certainly possible sources of virus which could then pass through the blood to the skeletal muscle where mutations occur that are then self limiting. It may be that these mutations are indeed short lived. This could explain the symptom of migrating myalgia.

As discussed elsewhere, one of the symptoms in M.E. and AOPVFS is that of tender muscles, particularly some have tender spots which come and go and move from place to place. This could reflect variable sites of muscle infection by enterovirus that lasts for a period of time and then disappears as the mutations self limit.

We also know that by studying muscle sections in other ways, that approximately only one fibre out of one hundred is infected with enterovirus sequences at any one time and that this infection does not seem to have any significant pathological effect on the other ninety nine per cent, so we certainly know that this muscle enterovirus infection is patchy and only affects very few fibres. Is it therefore the answer to the widespread global fatigue?

Epidemics

I think the epidemic form of AOPVFS must have the greatest argument for the potency of the initial virus infection, and for that of viral dose. There are a number of outbreaks in small institutions, where perhaps thirty or forty members of a school, army barracks or hospital go down with a virulent viral infection and many develop subsequent disease. Here, it is reasonable to suppose that the same strain of virus rapidly passed around in high doses of high virulence could be the answer as to the subsequent development of AOPVFS.

This situation also provides an argument against a genetic background, and against sex prevalence, because these epidemics have been found in army barracks, where the sufferers were all considered to be young, healthy men, and in boys' and girls' schools. Equally, there appears to be less ground for arguing stress factors or psychological predisposing influences. However, it may well be that the epidemic disorder is different aetiologically from the sporadic type.

To sum up, I feel that it is likely that the answers are going to be found in the virulence and the dose of the initial virus infection and, to a lesser extent, in predisposing, genetic and stress-related influences. It is going to be a few years yet before we get any further reasonable indicators to the epidemiology of this disease, and a lot more study is still required.

The ways in which we do not get M.E.

So far, the only viruses that we can find to link with M.E. and AOPVFS are persistent enteroviruses, reactivated EBV or, possibly, EBV as the aetiological agent. However, there is a group in which we can find no virology at all. This does not alter my viewpoint that M.E. and AOPVFS are virally precipitated immunological diseases, in which the precipitating virus may or may not persist.

I have heard many other suggestions as to the cause of the disease, most of which I consider to be quite unreasonable. However, it is worth discussing some of the alternative proposals, if only to dismiss them.

An M.E. virus?

The first one came up at the Annual General Meeting of the M.E. Association in 1986, when Dr Ramsay was asked to put forward the possibility of there being an M.E. virus – in other words, a particular virus, as yet undiscovered, that will cause M.E. I suggest that there is no such virus.

The sporadic cases account for by far the largest numbers of AOPVFS sufferers, and in these cases there is a close association with the enteroviruses. This is easily demonstrated by specific immunological and virological studies, which show the presence of a persistent enterovirus in a large proportion of both M.E. and AOPVFS patients. Using the new monoclonal antibodies, we are able to demonstrate evidence of persistent enterovirus antigen in the blood and muscle years after the initial infection. Enterovirus antibody can equally be shown.

There are cases where a whole family shares a proven enterovirus start. In some members the enterovirus disappears and they recover; one member goes on to develop AOPVFS, and the enterovirus persists. This demonstrates a close association between the disease and the enterovirus.

Even stronger evidence of persistent enterovirus is shown in the epidemic form. If one gets fifty people, all of whom have an enterovirus demonstrated in their blood, and all of whom are ill in the same initial outbreak, it would seem unreasonable to look for another virus as a causal agent.

More recently we have also been able to associate AOPVFS with an initial EBV infection, as shown by a positive Paul Bunnell or heterophile antibody test, and evidence of that virus remains in the blood as the patient continues to suffer. Other patients show an indication of EBV reactivation, but here I believe that something else has initiated this.

I do accept, however, that there is a theoretical possibility of there being a new, as yet unheard of virus that causes the problem. For the reasons that I have given, though, I think that it is extremely unlikely that we need to look for a new type of infecting organism which produces M.E. and M.E. alone.

M.E. from body fluids?

None of my AOPVFS patients suggested that they had developed their illness after receiving a blood transfusion, or any kind of injection containing blood products. There are a few people who develop their M.E. problem while in hospital having an operation. This is obviously an acute onset type as it can be pinpointed to the date of the operation but it may not be clear as to whether there was an acute viral onset.

Is M.E. contagious or infectious?

If, as I have already suggested, you can discount the possibility of there being a specific M.E. virus, leaving the disease as the result of at least two common viruses, then I believe that you cannot catch M.E.

My reasoning for the development of the disease is that the patient is exposed to a very common virus which, after initiating an infection, produces M.E. or AOPVFS because of an abnormal immunological response or virus penetration, or because of the virulence of that common virus.

In a sporadic case, a person will catch the enterovirus from a member of the family or from a casual contact; for the first few days of the infection the sufferer is acutely ill with a typical flu-like infection. He or she is also acutely infectious and may pass the virus on to anyone with whom he or she comes into contact. However, what he or she is passing on is the enterovirus, the Coxsackie B4 or the ECHO 19 – not AOPVFS or M.E. nor a predisposed genetic abnormality, nor a suppressed immunological status.

As to epidemics, if the virus itself is particularly virulent, then a whole group of people may be exposed to a large dose of virulent virus, passed on from one to another in the first few days of the infection. Since a causative factor may be the virulence of the virus and the dose received, many people may go on to develop AOPVFS as a result of the early infection. As the virulence of that virus is diminished by the introduction of defective interfering particles, other persons receiving it will experience a lower pathogenic effect and will suffer only a cold or flu with a normal recovery.

Now, let us consider whether the person who has developed M.E. as a result of their virus is infectious or contagious in any way.

In 40 per cent of sufferers we can demonstrate persistent enterovirus infection. Theoretically speaking, it would be possible for them to pass on their virus, although I think that this is unlikely. However, we can detect evidence of virus antigen in the blood, in the muscle, and we can recover whole infectious virus from the stool. It seems likely that those who have an intermittent sore throat are also shedding virus, but the virus from both the throat and the stool is heavily coated in antibody and therefore not infectious. It is this antibody binding that makes it so hard for us to find the virus in the laboratory; we have to take samples of stool, pour on acid, neutralize it and centrifuge it before we are able to discover it.

With regard to virus in the blood, this is certainly not infectious – it is virus VP1 antigen, i.e. only a bit of the capsule. So if you gave a pint of whole blood, you would not pass on anything, as far as we can establish.

As to the question of whether M.E. patients should be blood or organ donors, I believe that the worst thing that could happen would be that you could pass on your enterovirus infection, and the recipient of your blood or organ would simply develop a cold or flu. However, I do not really think that this is possible, because virus particle in the blood or the kidney has no evidence of being whole infective virus. Consequently, I see no harm in being a blood donor or an organ donor, although the Blood Transfusion Centre take a more cautious approach on this, believing it to be inadvisable.

If you have M.E. because of an abnormality in your white cell function, then I can see the possibility of being able to pass it on if you became a bone marrow donor. In that situation, you might be passing on your dysfunctional white cells and your inappropriate immune response, which could be the source of your own M.E. – but that, of course, is purely hypothetical.

The question of infectivity and EBV is slightly different. Twenty-five per cent of people with AOPVFS have evidence of reactivation of EBV in that they have an increased viral lytic cycle.

This could be purely due to the fact that they have a deficient white cell function, and the only problem lies within the bloodstream, with an increased turnover of infected B-cells and the production of virus. It is however possible that there is an increase in secretion of the Epstein Barr virus from infected mucus in the mouth. Healthy people secrete the virus to a greater or lesser extent, and this is a prime source of EBV generally; a person with an EBV related AOPVFS should therefore not consider themselves to be a leper, but might be secreting higher counts of infective virus from their saliva. Here again, they would not be passing on M.E. but the Epstein Barr virus, with the possibility of causing glandular fever.

Are M.E. and AOPVFS the same disease?

From my descriptions of M.E. and AOPVFS you can see that the symptoms of both are identical, while the virological and immunological abnormalities are very similar. The only real differences are in the stories of how the illness started and in their clinical progress. M.E. has a very slow, insidious onset and tends to chronicity rather than to improvement; AOPVFS has a very acute onset with more florid symptoms, shows more fluctuation and tends to improvement. This suggests that if they are the same disease, there are two different human responses to it.

If there is a method of differentiating between the clinical types and/or the virological response, then it is not immediately apparent to me. However, both James Mowbray and Jonathan Brostoff plan to take a group of AOPVFS and slow onset M.E. patients who show different virological responses – namely a positive VPI, reactivation of EBV or no virological abnormality detectable – and do an intensive study of them. It is clearly of great importance to us to find an answer because if there is a difference between M.E. and AOPVFS or between the enterovirus group and the reactivated EBV group, then it would give rise to the theoretical possibility of there being at least four different diseases, and possibly six – namely: M.E. plus VPI; M.E. plus EBV; M.E. plus ?; AOPVFS plus VPI; AOPVFS plus EBV; AOPVFS plus ?

Apart from the identical symptomatology, it is also noteworthy that exacerbating and improving factors are the same in both slow onset M.E. and AOPVFS. For example, intercurrent infection, trauma, operations, various foodstuffs, and alcohol make both groups worse; mental and physical rest, antidepressants and exclusion diets result in improvement. Further specific investigations also show similarities. The detailed results are still to be interpreted, but initially it would appear that both groups have the same skeletal muscle cellular RNA/DNA ratio deficiences. The same abnormalities can be seen in single muscle fibre EMG studies, and I suspect that examining skeletal muscle under the electron microscope histochemically and intracellularly for viral elements will also show the same result.

If slow onset M.E. and AOPVFS are indeed the same disease, my conclusion is that the virology is there by courtesy of the disease and is not the cause of it. Since one cannot detect either historically or by questioning what virology might be expected to be found in either slow onset M.E. or AOPVFS patients then the disease must have a different causative agent other than one specific virus.

The AOPVFS group are fit and well until they go down with a virus infection that they may share with other members of their family; the others get better, and they do not. This process suggests very strongly that the initial phenomenon is set off by an infective agent shared by that family which finds an abnormal immunological response in one member; that abnormal immunological response persists, and because it persists, it allows the virus to continue to be present.

When looking at patients who have VPI in their blood persistently, it is tempting to extrapolate that finding to suggest that their initial infection was an enterovirus but this may not be the case. It may be that the initial infection was a different virus which precipitated an abnormal immune response, and VPI is there as a consequence of that, possibly from a dormant carrier pool in the gastro-intestinal system. I have seen two particular groups of people in whom the virological findings suggest that this hypothesis could be correct.

One was a young husband and wife who had visited Italy, where within a short period both of them had gone down with a typical flu-like illness and subsequently developed a post viral type syndrome.

Nine months after this process had started the husband gave four positive VPI tests over a period of twelve weeks; the wife showed no evidence of VPI but there was virological evidence that suggested reactivation of EBV. I also looked at their neutralizing enterovirus antibody, at least as far as Coxsackie B was concerned; the husband had a fairly high titre to Coxsackie B3 of 1:512 and the wife did not. So this story suggests that they both acquired an M.E. syndrome at the same time from the same viral cause, although in one there was an enterovirus and in the other reactivation of EBV.

The second group was a family who all developed an acute flu-like illness which left the majority of them with an M.E. problem. The worst sufferers were the husband and wife, who displayed a persistent enterovirus; some of the children showed not only an enterovirus antigen, but also an enterovirus specific antibody. However, one of the elder children who also suffered from an M.E. syndrome showed no enterovirus antibody or antigen, but only a significant EBV effect.

The interpretation of these various virological findings is clearly of great importance. On the one hand it is possible that the virus itself of whatever type is causing the disorder, while on the other, the disorder allows the persistence of that virus. It is a chicken and egg situation that must be unravelled, because if viruses are causing the problem, we need to discover a way to kill them, whereas if they are not we would be wasting our time developing antiviral medications.

Holidays and vaccinations

Clearly, an AOPVFS or M.E. sufferer's holiday should be a quiet, relaxing one, with monitored physical effort. The ideal would be to lie in the warm sun by the side of a swimming pool for maximum mental and physical relaxation. Avoidance of extremes of temperature is advisable in as much as very hot or cold weather seems to exacerbate symptoms, but this is a matter of personal experience.

I do not know of any deleterious effects in the actual flight, although I cannot see how you are going to get round the possibility of a twelve hour delay at Gatwick. However, to minimize the problems, taking the journey in slow stages, perhaps with a night in a local hotel, would be a good idea.

As far as vaccinations are concerned, I feel it best, wherever possible, to avoid the following unless there is significant risk to health as a consequence: tetanus toxoid; typhoid; cholera; yellow fever. Those that can be taken without known problems are: polio (orally); hepatitis (intramuscularly); anti-malarial medication. However, just in case any of these upset you, arrange to have them well in advance to give you time to recover from any deleterious effects before your holiday.

12
LIVING WITH M.E. AND AOPVFS

The menstrual cycle

M.E. and AOPVFS mainly occur in young to middle-aged women, and the symptoms are invariably worsened premenstrually. This phenomenon is common to many medical problems, where there is either an exacerbation of a pre-existing premenstrual syndrome or it becomes evident for the first time.

This does not mean that premenstrual syndrome is necessarily a feature of M.E., but where present it can often be markedly improved by specific therapies. Medications that I have found helpful include diuretics, vitamin B6 and those with the natural hormone progesterone. There are other remedies both herbal and homeopathic and all of these possibilities should be discussed with your physician.

If the disease continues into later life, the M.E. and AOPVFS symptoms can become complicated with those of the menopause. Once again, my advice would be to seek specific medical opinion, as menopausal symptoms are very treatable.

M.E. and pregnancy

Having a baby is one of the fundamental human rights, and something that the vast majority of all married couples actively wish for. However, I have met several women with AOPVFS who have made a positive decision not to have a family because they feel they are too unwell to cope with looking after a child.

I feel that is wrong, and I always encourage people to have their family because their health tends to improve anyway, and with the correct management the problems after confinement can be minimized. I also believe that in the next few years we are going to have some effective treatment programmes.

It may be that those who make a conscious decision not to have a child lack adequate family support, which in this situation is clearly vitally important; and, obviously, some women are very unwell, and if they are unable to spend more than a few hours a day out of bed they must find contemplating a pregnancy difficult.

I have seen only eight patients through pregnancy and with that number I feel that I can give nothing more than the following simple overall view, without drawing any final significant conclusions.

Does it affect conception?

There is no evidence to suggest that the disease has any effect upon fertility and none of my patients had any difficulty in becoming pregnant.

Does it affect the baby?

Not as far as I am aware – M.E. is not a new disorder and there is no evidence that any foetal abnormalities that have occurred in the past have been associated with any specific fatigue syndrome.

Will the baby have M.E.?

No, I believe that it will not. I took blood samples from six of my patients and from their babies and there was no sign of any VPI antigen in the infants' blood. All eight babies have been fit and well, and have progressed normally.

Is M.E. inherited?

There is a possibility of a genetic predisposition to M.E. but as yet there is no proof of this. I have found, however, that the majority of people who develop the disease do not have any relatives with a similar disorder.

Does it affect the pregnancy?

The initial studies suggest that it does not. Having M.E. or AOPVFS does not seem to lead to any increase in miscarriage and pregnancies appear to be quite normal.

Confinement

The delivery of the baby will fatigue the mother more than it would a healthy person, and therefore assistance should be sought. Precisely what form this takes depends upon the advice given by the obstetrician – it is important to discuss the various aspects of the disease with him or her so that he or she can provide adequate support. It may be that a forceps delivery or, in more severe cases, a Caesarean section is advisable.

We do not know at this stage whether any of the uterine functions during delivery are affected. The majority of the physical effort of delivery is produced by the uterus with added push provided by the mother, and it is the latter aspect that is the tiring factor in the delivery.

Aftercare

It is likely that there will be an exacerbation of symptoms during the confinement, but they should not result in long-term problems. My patients have not suffered any notable deterioration, although several members of the M.E. Association report significant setbacks. However, even if there is such a setback recovery will be the rule, and with the support of the nursing staff within the hospital, perhaps a few extra days' rest after the delivery, and adequate help at home from midwife, family and husband, the problems should be minimized.

What about new symptoms?

The symptomatology of M.E. and AOPVFS is extensive and diverse. After the initial disease onset has settled and the pattern of symptoms has been adjusted to, what happens if new problems arise?

Generally speaking, any new symptoms should be investigated appropriately, and if any results are positive that medical problem should then be treated. Do not forget that having M.E. does not disallow you from developing acute appendicitis, so do not ignore new afflictions – discuss them with your doctor.

I can only hope that he or she is understanding and patient because many new symptoms that occur are associated with the disease process. Meanwhile, old ones disappear. The whole disease process is one of natural fluctuation.

Body weight and M.E.

I have observed that the weight of M.E. patients seems to fluctuate quite markedly. Some notice that unless they eat frequently they feel dizzy, faint and unwell, and that this is alleviated by food, consequently they put on weight. Others, however, are troubled by indigestion or nausea to such an extent that they are put off food, and then they find they lose a lot of weight. This can become such a problem that anorexia can set in, with loss of muscle bulk and sometimes cessation of normal menstrual cycle.

Both of these extremes of normal body weight should be avoided wherever possible. Being overweight when suffering from M.E. is clearly a disadvantage, as carrying around a few extra pounds is only going to compound the problem of excessive muscular fatigueability. On the other hand, significant loss of weight and anorexia must put the body's natural capability for recovery in jeopardy. The ideal weight, then, is neither too fat nor too thin, but slightly on the thinner side of normal.

13

TREATMENTS

Every M.E. Association Newsletter contains stories of remedies that have helped or even cured some poor soul suffering from this horrendous disease. The national newspapers ran a story of how someone who had been suffering from M.E. for two or three years was cured in three weeks by an anti-Parkinsonian drug. The Charing Cross Hospital claims significant improvement from sleep therapy; the Sleep Laboratory at St Mary's Hospital suggests that not breathing in enough oxygen at night either causes or significantly contributes to the symptomatology; psychiatrists offer specific antidepressants; one physician told me that he thought he could cure 70 per cent of post viral syndrome in three weeks with EPD (Enzyme Potentiated Desensitization); the Institute of Neurological Sciences in Glasgow has used oil of evening primrose and expounded its benefits, as has a neurological institution in Coventry.

These possibilities are put forward by standard medical bodies. When you venture into the more peripheral fields, the treatments become a little more arcane. Homoeopathic practitioners abound, although they do not claim significant cures. Allergy treatment centres are expensive, indeed, a course of treatment may run into five figures. Candida diets and Nystatin are very popular as an antidote to antibiotics, which allow the yeasts that infest the bowel to multiply. Bio-ergonomics machines imported from Germany measure some strange electrical activity, while another machine takes the power from parts of the body and diagnoses allergy. Some people have their mercury amalgam fillings taken out and replaced with composites, but the expected cure does not seem to come about.

I used to be amazed at the number of vitamin and mineral supplements that Americans took, but I must admit that the M.E. sufferer is coming a good second best. Most people do not see any harm in taking vitamins and minerals, and there has recently been some evidence that lack of vitamins prevents schoolchildren achieving their expected learning capabilities, so there is a flourishing trade in these supplements, particularly in intravenous vitamin C. I cannot see why the latter should be more efficacious than vitamin C taken by any other means, and it is certainly more expensive. It is also suggested that zinc deficiency may be implicated in M.E., so many people take supplements of this in the hope of improvement.

I get at least one letter per week telling me how this new substance or that new treatment has cured somebody with M.E. and my attitude is one of scepticism. Consequently, I must apply the same objectivity to my own treatment. Seven years ago I started using intramuscular pooled human gamma globulin, and I was impressed by the number of people who showed an improvement. However, I stopped using it about three years ago, not because this improvement stopped, but because I was acutely aware of the fact that I was giving a remedy which was not provably efficient, and we needed to do a double blind trial in order to find out beyond doubt whether this substance worked or not. I currently use very little gamma globulin in treating post viral syndrome, supplying it only to those patients who have used it for some time and profess to feel better for it.

I can well understand, however, this mushrooming alternative therapy approach. When patients come to see me or any other doctor specializing in post viral syndrome only to be told that there is nothing that can be done, they must go away very disheartened. The prospect of being ill for possibly several years to come must be terrifying, and the need to find something that will help becomes very strong. Thus the M.E. sufferer will do the rounds of various alternative practitioners in an attempt to find the cure.

It is psychologically better to be busy and to be doing something that does not work, rather than sitting back and doing nothing at all, which also does not work. I therefore do not disapprove of people trying any remedy, whether it be scientifically proven or not, as long as it does not fall into the category of being dangerous or, alternatively, unreasonably expensive. However, I believe that we need to find out the cause of the disease before developing treatment programmes around informed medical evidence. Until we do, I see little prospect of a cure, and I suggest to all of those practising alternative remedies that they should undertake scientifically controlled and medically accepted double blind trials that will stand up to scrutiny as being a provable efficacious programme. Until then, I will reject all claims that one particular treatment or another works.

AOPVFS is a disease which can extend into years. It is a naturally fluctuating one, with exacerbations and remissions, and it tends to improve; it also tends, with increasing time, to chronicity. Within this type of disease process, of which there are several, multiple sclerosis and rheumatoid arthritis to name but two, there tends to be a tremendously strong placebo effect. It is a scientifically proven fact that if you give a group of chronic sufferers a particular treatment 30 per cent of them will feel better regardless of what you use. This is the placebo effect, and it is as evident in AOPVFS as in any other disease.

It is, unfortunately, possible that an alternative approach may do more harm than good. I recall a young girl who was made seriously ill by a diet that was given to her by a homeopathic practitioner. She had AOPVFS and was virtually bed-bound, and had been for some considerable time. Everything had been tried, and her parents, who are very sensible, intelligent folk, put her on a particularly stringent diet on the advice of the practitioner. They went on with this diet for some six months, until one day the patient started to develop chest discomfort and shortness of breath. She was admitted to hospital with heart failure; she had developed beri-beri because her diet had not included adequate amounts of vitamins. She had also become anorexic, her periods had stopped and other secondary catabolic processes had set in whereby she had lost muscle bulk, and other body tissues.

On the other side of the fence, I have seen patients who have been placed on various medications by their GP and who have developed a habituation to the drug they were taking. I have in mind two particular female patients who, because they had been diagnosed as having an anxiety state rather than the organic disease that AOPVFS is, had been placed on the tranquillizer Ativan. The AOPVFS had got better in both cases, but they were still suffering from horrendous psychological symptomatology, the side effects, I believe, of Ativan addiction, and trying to get them off this medication proved to be extremely difficult. Consequently, I am not suggesting that bad treatments stem only from alternative practitioners; my view is that all medications and treatment programmes should be used wisely and carefully.

Optimising your capability of improvement

While there is no cure for AOPVFS and M.E., there is no doubt that one can aid one's body to make its own improvement. The most important single aspect of this whole problem is that of disease management and this includes caring for one's body in a global fashion and helping the immune system to deal with things as best it can.

I am not aware of any commonly available substance that is proven to act as an immuno-stimulant, although there are many therapeutic regimes offered by many branches of medicine. However, sensible suggestions would of course include stopping smoking, cutting down on alcohol, eating a sensible diet and avoiding preservatives, colouring agents or multi-processed foods. Don't take medications unless they have been fully discussed with a physician.

Relaxation, meditation and related therapies

There is little doubt in my mind that stress in its various forms has a part to play in the causative factors of AOPVFS, but it is much more difficult to assess in slow onset M.E. Once the disease is established, however, many of the symptoms that occur in both groups are associated with tension or anxiety both physical and mental; muscle tension, spasm and pain are commonplace.

The understanding and management of these problems and their improvement with various treatments offers the best area of therapeutic success among all the symptoms noted in M.E. I recommend that when searching for relaxation therapy the patient should try several types to find which is most appropriate to him or her.

There is a wide range of options, some of which are available through the NHS, although the majority are found elsewhere. Specific relaxation can be most helpful and it is often something that needs to be taught, as people can frequently be very tense even when they think they are relaxed. This is available by referral by your GP to the psychological services found at the majority of the larger local hospitals. Relaxation classes can be a continued support; they usually consist of a dozen or so sessions, either with a psychologist or, in smaller groups, with a psychiatrist. Individual tapes for relaxation can be made in such sessions and less tailor-made cassettes can be bought, or even borrowed from some lending libraries.

Other types of specific relaxation can be found in yoga and various meditation classes, usually not found within the health service. Advertisements for them can usually be found in local papers, in libraries and in health food shops.

For non-structured forms of relaxation, try passive physiotherapy, saunas, massage etc. Again this is a matter of individual choice, as some might find a sauna makes them worse not better.

Chronic anxiety and tension can produce an alteration in immune response and it has been suggested that antidepressants, relaxation therapy and meditation improve immune regulation. I am not at all sure, however, that this would contribute much to curing M.E.

Sleep, hyperventilation and sleep apnoea

It is the norm to find quite marked disturbances of sleep in both slow onset M.E. and AOPVFS, but more so in the latter, especially in the initial acute phase. Patients find that no matter how exhausted they are their mind remains hyperactive; when sleep finally comes it is restless and unrewarding, leaving them as tired in the morning as they were when they went to bed. Dreams, and often nightmares, are vivid and are frequently remembered in colour.

Dealing with this sleep problem is important, because obtaining rest, both physically and mentally, at night will provide much more mental and physical strength during the day. Fortunately, this is one area of symptomatology that can be greatly improved.

The first remedies to try are simple ones such as a warm milky drink, a relaxing bath, relaxation tapes or some form of meditation. If these fail move on to medication, both standard and alternative. Of the former type, I dislike hypnotics such as benzodiazepines which tend to be habituating, favouring instead the sedative tricyclic or quadracyclic antidepressants (see pp. 217–9).

Achieving a more relaxed and rewarding sleep will maximize your capability of recovering, or at least feeling better in the interim.

Sleep apnoea

Researchers at St Mary's Hospital, Paddington, have suggested that some patients with M.E. are suffering from sleep apnoea.

Sleep apnoea is the slowing and possibly brief cessation of breathing during sleep. There may be as long as five to fifteen seconds between breaths and this occurs intermittently all night, which means that by morning the patient may have lost anything from several minutes to an hour of normal breathing. During that time, the oxygen level in the blood goes down, and so the patient wakes in the morning feeling groggy, headachey, and generally unwell. A preliminary study on patients with M.E. has linked them with this phenomenon and giving them oxygen during the night appeared to alleviate many of the symptoms. This still requires further study, and an extensive research programme has been put forward.

My initial comment on this is that there was no disease definition in the initial cases and, as the perception of M.E. can be markedly different from one observer to another, I am not sure what clinical group was involved.

Hyperventilation syndrome

In August 1988, a group of workers at Charing Cross Hospital suggested that AOPVFS was caused by, or at least the majority of the symptoms were attributable to, hyperventilation syndrome. They found that by teaching correct breathing techniques and including prolonged sleep, the patients' health could be improved.

If you breathe too deeply or too quickly or both, you are said to be hyperventilating. For any given physical state there is a specific amount of energy required, and this is obtained by a process of cellular metabolism requiring oxygen. This metabolism of food is equivalent to it being 'burnt'. During this process energy is released, oxygen is consumed and carbon dioxide is produced. If you do virtually nothing, as in normal sleep, the amount of energy required is minimal, but there is a baseline tick-over of oxygen being breathed in and carbon dioxide being puffed out. If your activity rises, as would be the case in running, and the energy requirements are higher, the oxygen consumption is raised and the carbon dioxide produced is correspondingly increased.

To achieve this, you breathe more deeply and rapidly, but this increased rate and depth of breathing is in response to a bodily need for increased oxygen requirement and carbon dioxide output. Consequently, nothing untoward happens from a clinical point of view, except that you might feel a little puffed. If, on the other hand, you increase your breathing depth and rate unnecessarily then something quite different happens. Oxygen intake into the lungs will be increased, but as your blood is probably 98 per cent saturated with oxygen anyway, the amount going into the bloodstream is hardly affected. However, the amount of carbon dioxide breathed out is increased, and quite markedly so.

The amount of carbon dioxide in the blood is normally controlled at very specific levels; indeed, its presence is critical because it forms the basis of the degree of acidity of the blood. Carbon dioxide forms carbonic acid in the serum of the blood, and the acidity of the blood has a Ph of 6.7, a level that is maintained plus or minus 0.1 all day, every day. If you start to breathe off carbon dioxide from the blood without producing more by physical activity, then the acidity of your blood diminishes, and the Ph will rise. When your blood becomes more alkaline the calcium which is found freely circulating in the blood drops, disappearing from the bloodstream.

This unbalanced physiological state, known as tetany, leads to an increase in spontaneous nerve conduction and a diminution in muscle contraction. This initially results in pins and needles in the hands and feet, followed by pins and needles around the face, especially the mouth, and then pins and needles all over. One feels faint, headachey, weak and lethargic, symptoms which are found in AOPVFS. This unnecessary overbreathing is called hyperventilation syndrome.

There are many observers of M.E. in all its types who feel that hyperventilation has a part to play in the production of symptomatology. This may be true but, in my experience, that part is quite small. I certainly feel that hyperventilation is not implicated in the development of M.E. and even if you cure it the best you will find is an improvement in the more minor M.E. symptoms.

People with M.E. often experience anxiety and this may lead to hyperventilation, so if you suffer from some of the symptoms mentioned above, especially the pins and needles and light-headedness, then you should consider looking at your own breathing quality. The best form of treatment here is to consult a physiotherapist who has an interest in hyperventilation and to go on to a re-breathing course to learn how to breathe more sensibly.

Sleep apnoea and hyperventilation are two extremes of a normal breathing pattern. If they truly are part of the disease process of M.E. then it would not seem unreasonable to suggest that they could be due to an alteration of the breathing 'centre'. Deep inside your brain, literally between your ears, is an area of brain tissue that monitors the quantity of oxygen and the acidity and amount of carbon dioxide present in your blood, and as a result of that determines how much your breathe. I am certain that there are many areas of brain tissue affected by the M.E. process, and it may be that the breathing centre is one of them.

Sedatives and antidepressants

Sedatives

On the whole, I really cannot think of any good reason why sedatives should be helpful. Patients with AOPVFS are fatigued and giving them tranquillizers is surely simply going to compound that distressing problem. The majority of patients that I have seen who have been on sedatives have been prescribed them because the diagnosis has been a psychiatric one; their GPs have aimed to reduce their sleep disturbance, anxiety and panic attacks by prescribing an anxiolytic medication, the majority of which are found in the group of drugs known as benzodiazepines.

The most famous of the benzodiazepines is diazepam (Valium). This medication was brought out in the 1960s as the answer for all anxieties – 'mother's little helper'. Since that time many other benzodiazepines have been developed to be more specific towards anxiety or towards induction of sleep. These are the two major functions of the benzodiazepines.

Benzodiazepines that are advocated for anxiety include: Diazepam (Valium, Alupram, Atensine, Diazemuls, Evacalm, Solis, Stesolid, Tensium); ketazolam (Anxon); lorazepam (Ativan, Almazine); clobazam (Frisium); bromazepam (Lexotan); chlordiazepoxide (Librium); medazepam (Nobrium); oxazepam (Oxanid); alprazolam (Xanax). Benzodiazepines that are more specific towards sleep induction are: flurazepam (Dalmane); loprazolam (Dormonoct); triazolam (Halcion); nitrazepam (Mogadon); lormetazepam (Lormetazepam); temazepam (Normison); flunitrazepam (Rohypnol).

These anti-anxiety and sleep induction medications, of which I have named probably about half, all work in the same way and they all have the same drawbacks; they are addictive and they sedate anxiety but do not lift mood. The benzodiazepines should be restricted to short-term use, somewhere between two and four weeks. Those that are used for induction of sleep are, after only a very short period of time, very hard to stop taking without having weeks of sleeplessness. Withdrawal symptoms can be very startling and can produce exacerbation of all of the symptoms of AOPVFS, so much so that patients often find them impossible to manage without.

Benzodiazepines are a double-edged sword in the treatment of AOPVFS because they are also muscle relaxants, and so might help as far as muscle spasms and pain are concerned. However, they make the weakness and fatigue worse, and when they are withdrawn there is an increase in muscle spasm and pain as a side-effect.

I feel therefore that the benzodiazepines should *not* be used in AOPVFS except in the shortest of courses to help the patient face a situation which will cause acute anxiety. Apart from the problems mentioned above, it is a possibility that some of the symptomatology of AOPVFS is due to abnormal functioning of the central nervous system transmittors, and the fact that benzodiazepines are believed to have a specific effect upon one of those neuro-transmittors makes for another convincing argument against their use.

If the patient does require medication to reduce anxiety I feel that some of the beta-blockers are more appropriate. These were developed to regulate the production of adrenaline and noradrenaline so as to reduce the heart rate and lower the blood pressure. One of the effects of over-stimulation of adrenaline is to produce anxiety, so some of the agitation and phobic symptomatology of AOPVFS can be helpfully controlled in some cases by the use of medications like propranolol, whether in short-acting form or longer-acting time capsules. Individual doses should be tailor-made for the patient involved, and as there are side-effects and contra-indications in some cases the use of beta-blockers must be carefully discussed with the doctor.

Antidepressants

Patients with AOPVFS or M.E. do tend to improve by taking antidepressants, but again this is an improvement in symptomatology, not a movement towards a cure.

Once a patient has obtained a diagnosis of AOPVFS or M.E. and it is understood that this is organically based, he or she should not be in any way concerned when the physician offers him or her an antidepressant. These drugs are safe and non-addictive, and they are used for several different reasons. The benefits they offer include reducing anxiety; lifting mood; reducing emotional lability;

relieving depression, both primary and reactive; alleviating phobic symptoms; inducing sleep; and calming irritable bowel syndrome. However, while I advocate antidepressants of various types, they do have side-effects, and I would not wish to suggest that they are a panacea.

Among the more important side-effects of the tricyclic and quadracyclic antidepressants are the following drawbacks. Some people simply cannot tolerate them, so a very small test dose should be taken initially to see if the patient feels unwell. They sometimes cause blurring of vision, and this can be a problem in those who already have sight problems. They also tend to lead to a dry mouth. Sedation can be quite marked, and some patients have a problem in waking up in the morning, although this tends to wear off after a week or so. If it continues a less sedative type of antidepressant should be considered, and there are a variety of those. Palpitation is not uncommon when using antidepressants, and since this is found in AOPVFS they might lead to an increase in heart irregularity; this could be settled with beta-blockers, if the beneficial effects of the antidepressants outweigh the side-effects. Bowel mobility is reduced, causing constipation, and the appetite is increased, so the patient may put on weight.

The tricyclic antidepressants work by being absorbed into the central nervous system, where they prevent the re-uptake of some of the neuro-transmittors, specifically noradrenaline and serotonin, thereby increasing the levels of those chemicals at the neuro-transmittor junction (see p. 230–31). The complete mode of action of the tricyclic antidepressants remains obscure, but it is believed that patients who have a depressive illness have a generalized lowering of neuro-transmittor levels.

Examples of sedative tricyclic antidepressants are: trimipramine (Surmontil); doxepin (Sinequan); dopthiepin (Prothiaden); amitriptyline (Tryptizol). Antidepressants with a less sedative effect include: nortriptyline (Aventyl, Allegron); clomipramine (Anafranil); protriptyline (Concordin); butriptyline (Evadyne).

The quadracyclic antidepressants have probably the same type of pharmacological action as the tricyclics; some are believed to increase the release of neuro-transmittors as well as blocking their re-uptake. Their side effects tend to be slightly less than the tricyclic antidepressants, and they are certainly not as sedative. I favour the quadracyclics out of all the antidepressants. Examples are: triazolopyridine (Molipaxin); maprotiline hydrochloride (Ludiomil).

I also find the monoamine oxidase inhibitors (MAOI) group very helpful. They tend to be rather neutral in their effect, being neither particularly stimulating nor sedative, but some patients do find them sufficiently stimulating that if they are already suffering sleep disturbance they should avoid this group.

These antidepressants cause some dietary problems in that foods containing a lot of monoamines should be abstained from. These include meat extracts such as Oxo and Bovril, Marmite, various gravy cubes, cheese and some wines. Nevertheless, the monoamine oxidase inhibitors, which include isocarboxazid (Marplan) and phenelzine (Nardil), still have a valuable role to play in the management of M.E. and AOPVFS.

Of all these psychotropic medications I would on the whole eschew the sedatives and tranquillizers and would prefer to see a greater use of the antidepressants. The latter can be used in conjunction with other anxiolytic medications such as the beta-blockers and should be adjusted to suit each patient, using both the expertise of the physician and trial and error. One antidepressant may agree with one patient much better than another, so do not hesitate to try different varieties until you find one that helps you.

Pain killers

Pain is unfortunately quite a common problem in AOPVFS and M.E. and, while affecting various parts of the body, it is mainly found in four large areas: myalgia (muscle pains); arthralgia (joint pains); neuralgia (nerve pains); and headache.

Both AOPVFS and M.E. are unfortunately likely to be long illnesses and therefore finding appropriate medication that is both effective and safe is a matter of importance. Consequently, the suggestions that I am making here should be discussed at length with your own physician, as there are contra-indications to many remedies.

The first consideration is whether any medication should be taken at all, or whether simply understanding the disease process and its management might not be the best analgesic. Some non-specific remedies have been suggested elsewhere, including relaxation therapy and meditation, and other non-medication approaches such as acupuncture and physiotherapy can also be tried. These approaches have very personal responses, and a remedy that is effective in one patient may not be so in another.

If none of them are sufficiently effective then you should consider medication but, even where this is relatively innocuous, never exceed the recommended dose or the recommended length of treatment without further advice from your GP.

There are a lot of preparations available over the counter without prescription, but even these, when taken over a long period of time, can cause significant medical problems. For instance, continuing courses of paracetamol, which can be bought under a variety of brand names, can be deleterious to the liver and kidney. Aspirin, while it can be effective, can lead to chronic gastro-intestinal irritation and bleeding, causing anaemia and possibly intestinal ulceration. Other easily acquired non-steroidal anti-inflammatories (NSAIs) such as ibuprofen have the same side-effects as aspirin, added to which they can cause specific disorders of the blood.

Pain relief must therefore be approached with care, and with an enquiring mind. Experimenting with smaller doses of various combinations of medication may bring more effective relief than a large dose of one substance.

The major medications

Analgesics

Pure analgesia is specifically the reduction of pain. Nobody is certain at what level most analgesics act, but probably the major function is that of altering the production of pain-stimulating chemicals produced by cells within the brain itself and locally at the site from where the pain originates.

Pain killers include:

Aspirin: Probably one of the oldest substances known to give pain relief, it comes in several forms. If it is going to be taken over any considerable period of time, I would prefer the enteric coated variety (E/C), such as Nu-seals, where the aspirin substance is coated in a further set of compounds which delay its absorption until it reaches the small bowel, thus minimizing the irritative property that it so frequently has in the stomach. For occasional use, choose the soluble forms of aspirin, which are much cheaper.

During long-term use, blood tests should be performed in order to ensure that anaemia or blood problems do not occur. If indigestion becomes a significant problem, the aspirin should be taken with food and/or alkalis and if this does not clear it up, the medication should be discontinued and probably medical advice sought.

Paracetamol: A very popular, simple pain killer available in several proprietary brands, which, when taken in the prescribed dose, do not cause many problems. There are also combination medications containing paracetamol, some of which are available over the counter, but the majority, especially the stronger ones, are only available by prescription.

Stronger analgesics – all of which are available only on prescription – include Fortral, DF118, and Sublingual Temgesic. Some of these have problems with habituation and so regular usage is not advisable; it also diminishes their efficiency. Take these medications only in short courses, or even in single doses.

Anti-inflammatories

By far the largest and most commonly prescribed pain relievers belong to a group collectively known as the non-steroidal anti-inflammatories (the NSAIs). They were developed because some of the most potent anti-inflammatory medications ever discovered belonged to the group of steroids, which, while being efficient in removing inflammation, have potentially serious side-effects. In any event, steroids should not be considered in the treatment of muscle aches and pains, or any other kind of pain experienced in AOPVFS, as there is no evidence of any inflammatory process. So if there is no inflammation, why consider the non-steroidal anti-inflammatories?

The answer is that this particular group of drugs, apart from being anti-inflammatory, are also markedly analgesic, being in many cases more potently so than some of the stronger pure analgesics such as DF118. They were mainly developed for the treatment of the inflammatory arthritic diseases such as rheumatoid arthritis and, to a lesser extent, osteo-arthritis. There are many to choose from, including: ibuprofen (Brufen, Ebufac, Fenbid); oxicam (Feldene); proponic acid (Fenopron, Froben); salicylate (Dolobid).

Ibuprofen was one of the first to be developed, and is available directly over the counter. These medications vary in both their anti-inflammatory and their analgesic properties and where one may work another might not, so it is worthwhile trying several before considering the group as a whole to be ineffective.

There are several well known side-effects and they include indigestion, dizziness and gastro-intestinal bleeding and upset. These drugs should not be taken by anyone suffering from gastric ulcers or kidney trouble. The NSAI group can be taken in combination with analgesics or other drugs to enhance their analgesic or anti-inflammatory effect.

Muscle relaxants

Diazepam: I am not at all happy about the prolonged use of benzodiazepines, (see pp. 215–7), but in certain exceptional circumstances diazepam has a place. Apart from being a sedative, it is an effective muscle relaxant so if one of the major symptoms is that of muscle spasm and twitching diazepam may be an answer. However, it should always be used in the smallest possible doses, and as infrequently as possible to avoid habituation.

Meprobamate: This is particularly effective with the analgesics, but habituation is again a noticeable effect.

Antidepressants

Both the quadracyclic and tricyclic antidepressants are helpful in the reduction of pain by altering the perception of the sensory input into the central nervous system. The sedative variety particularly also have muscle relaxant properties.

All of the above medications can be tried in various permutations, under medical advice, for the treatment of myalgia and arthralgia. When it comes to headache, there are a great number of specific medications available apart from those mentioned above, too many to go into in any detail here. While the headache itself is not typically migrainous, advice from migraine specialist bodies can be helpful.

'Shooting pains', which are less common but can be really quite severe when they do occur, are often of a neuralgia type. Again, there are specific remedies available, such as carbamazepine (Tegretol); sodium valproate (Epilim); clonidine hydrochloride (Dixarit); pizotifen (Sanomigen).

Mineral supplementation

A patient suffering from M.E. will usually have had routine biochemical screening done on at least one occasion, probably initially by a GP and certainly at any specialized out-patient clinic.

The type of investigation done would be what is referred to as a 10 channel SMAC. This includes the analysis of several of the major minerals and electrolytes found in the blood plasma, but there would not be, unless specifically requested, specialized investigations for the trace elements. Consequently, zinc and magnesium are not normally tested for except by specialized laboratories, usually on a private basis.

Other workers in the field of M.E. have told me that they frequently find quite significant lowering of zinc and magnesium in patients and they therefore recommend replacement therapy. Zinc is a vital co-enzyme and magnesium is of fundamental importance in the normal biochemical processes in the production of power within muscles: as they are water-soluble substances and not likely to be 'over-stored' within the body's tissues I see no harm in taking supplements. The recommended dosage is 30mg of zinc a day, in one dose, and 100mg of magnesium twice a day. If you do not notice any improvement after a month or so, stop taking them and see if any regression occurs. I cannot see the point in continuing to take substances unless they do some good even if they apparently do no harm.

Food and chemical intolerance

Food and chemical intolerance is an area of medicine which is even more controversial than AOPVFS itself. A large proportion of the M.E. Association members believe that all the answers lie within the allergy field, but I am quite prepared to state that in my view allergies and AOPVFS have little, if anything, to do with each other. However, should convincing evidence arise to the contrary, I am prepared to change my present stance.

Patients frequently tell me that some chemicals or foods make their symptoms worse, especially those associated with the gastro-intestinal tract and the central nervous system, including depression, anxiety, sleep disturbance and difficulties with concentration. These problems clearly need further identification and understanding.

I would be prepared to bet that everybody has an intolerance to something, while some have a true allergy. I myself have a relative intolerance to various types of alcohol – if I drink too much red wine or port I come out in blotches, develop a migrainous headache and start to wheeze. However, I do not identify that as an allergy but more a chemical intolerance to some of the substances found in red wine and port, probably the monoamines and the pressor chemicals (see p. 186). Whisky I can tolerate very happily. I cannot eat mussels or red and green peppers, but I am sure everybody has similar problems. We all have something that we can't eat or drink because it upsets us, it gives us nightmares, migrainous headaches, indigestion or something else, and I perceive this whole problem of chemical and food intolerance as being an increased sensitivity to these various substances.

It seems likely that we have a sensitivity to a majority fo foodstuffs which, when we are fit and healthy, does not cause any particular difficulties. In the AOPVFS sufferer, that intolerance is either heightened or the body's resistance to it is lowered. Many M.E. patients dislike perfumes, and develop nausea and headaches if exposed to cooking smells. I suggest that this may be associated with disturbance in neuro-transmittor levels (see p. 229–30).

The relatively small chemical molecules found in such odours are absorbed into the bloodstream via the lungs very quickly, and they have a very rapid effect, measured in minutes rather than hours, as do chemicals that require very little in the way of digestion, such as those found in tea and coffee. The same applies to strong-flavoured foods and the chemicals contained therein – strong cheese, onions and the like – and patients can easily identify the foodstuffs that make them feel worse, and so avoid them.

When you move on to some of the other food intolerance possibilities which involve long-chained molecules such as are found in proteins, the story is not so easy to interpret. Some patients have told me that they think milk upsets them, and so they have excluded it from their diet and felt slightly better for it, but they could not seem to identify other substances easily. I believe this is because the metabolism of such complex proteins is a lot slower.

As an example, let us take beef and its protein constituent. A protein is made up of basic building blocks called amino-acids. There are many of these, and they are arranged within beef in a very specific order which is not found in any other protein. They are grouped into peptides, which may consist of five, ten or fifty amino-acids. These peptides are then grouped together in chains called poly-peptides, and the poly-peptide chain forms a protein.

So the protein of beef is a unique structure which, when eaten, is broken down by enzymes within the stomach, duodenum and small bowel. The protein is absorbed, not in the basic building blocks of amino-acids, but in the smaller chains of poly-peptides. Within the human body peptides and poly-peptides are used biochemically and neurologically in a great number of reactions; some peptides are active neuro-transmittors and the intake of a pharmacologically active substance could aggravate the symptomatology in a person suffering from M.E.

Exclusion diet for AOPVFS and M.E.

To drink:

> Bottled mineral water
>   (any type)
> and/or
> 7 Up (not the diet form)

To eat:

Either: Fresh chicken, roasted
             (including chicken liver and
             offal), nil in it or on it
Or: White fish (any type) boiled in water*
And: Salt and pepper
And: Rice (any type)*
And: Brassica (cabbage and family)*
             Broccoli
             Brussels sprouts
             Cauliflower
             Cabbage
             Kohl rhabi
And: Any fruit not eaten in the last six
             months

*To be boiled in mineral water.

I can thus see a reasonable explanation for M.E. patients to experience increased chemical and food intolerance and the only way to pinpoint which substances are causing the problem is to try a total exclusion diet. There are several books devoted to this subject and I am offering only simple guidelines which I have used with some degree of success.

Nothing is allowed that is not on that list, not even medications. The 7 Up may seem a surprising inclusion, but its ingredients appear to be remarkably uncomplicated, consisting of water, sugar and extracts of lime and lemon with carbon dioxide. Fresh lemon and lime and other citrus fruits, either eaten whole or squeezed for a drink, are also allowed. The chicken is simply roasted in the oven and eaten hot or cold; the rice can be of any variety as long as it is not processed, and may be cooked with salt and bottled water or stir-fried in chicken fat. The vegetables should ideally be fresh, but frozen ones are acceptable. These also should be cooked in bottled water with salt to taste or stir-fried with the chicken fat. The fruit should be fresh for preference or, failing that, frozen; processed fruit will not do.

This diet should be adhered to for some ten days. I accept that it is a little boring but it is enough to sustain life, and if any significant food intolerance is contributing to the symptomatology the patient would expect to feel better after that period of time. Any improvement is most likely to be found in sleep pattern, depression, concentration, headaches and the gastro-intestinal symptoms of bloated stomach, flatulence, and the irritable bowel syndrome. Such improvement may be only slight, but I estimate that some 20 per cent of patients note a significant alleviation of their symptoms, enough to warrant going on to the second stage – the reintroduction of other food substances.

One uncomplicated new food can then be added to the diet every three days, in order of personal preference. For instance, if the patient wants a cup of tea this is allowable, as long as it does not contain milk. I suggest the continued exclusion of beef, all dairy products and all wheat products, as I have found that if patients are sensitive to any foodstuffs it tends to be one or other or all of these.

There are many specialists in this field and if food intolerance is a problem then it is best to seek expert help. However, although dietary advice is very important, I do not feel that it leads to any kind of cure, only to a generalized improvement; whether or not this improvement facilitates the natural recovery which normally occurs, I do not know. I have heard claims made by practitioners in dietary advice that I believe are unacceptable and should be taken with a large pinch of salt!

Hypoglycaemia

I have no precise figures as to how many of my patients have complained of hypoglycaemia, but I would estimate somewhere in the region of 5 per cent. The symptoms are interesting in that they may well point to food sensitivity.

When the patient becomes hungry the level of blood sugar drops and he or she starts to feel dizzy, faint and nervous. This can be immediately cured by eating, although the patient unfortunately tends to crave for sweet things – pastries, cakes, chocolates and the like – which cause the symptoms to recur more swiftly than unsweetened and unprocessed foods.

It has been suggested that in M.E. and AOPVFS there is some kind of abnormal glucose metabolism and an abnormal energy pathway, but most of those with this hypoglycaemic type of symptomatology show, when investigated, quite normal blood sugars. This can be tested by a glucose tolerance test, which involves starving the patient overnight and taking a blood sample some ten hours later. The patient then drinks a strong solution of glucose and its absorption and the speed with which it falls off over the next three or four hours is measured by taking frequent blood tests.

These hypoglycaemic symptoms can result in people putting on weight because they need to eat frequently and the temptation is to eat 'empty' calories, such as chocolates, sweets and starch. It is infinitely preferable to choose unsweetened biscuits such as oatcakes for snacks and, for meals, high-fibre unprocessed foods. This ameliorates the problem of weight gain and of fluctuating blood sugar levels.

There is as yet no explanation for the hypoglycaemic symptoms in patients who give a normal glucose tolerance test. It has been suggested that people who are sensitive to various foods get a type of withdrawal effect when they do not eat them, and also that this type of symptomatology is related to candida infestation. I cannot accept the latter theory, but I have to admit that I have no explanation to offer.

The alcohol problem

It is remarkable how people with AOPVFS develop an intolerance of alcohol. In the initial acute phase, general illness and malaise discourage the desire to drink alcohol anyway, but even after some degree of recovery the patients find that alcoholic drinks make them ill.

I became aware of this fact very early in my work on this disorder, because a large number of people made this point and it was certainly borne out by the study, which showed a true figure of 92 per cent avoiding alcohol. I found this very interesting, as there are not many medical conditions where patients spontaneously stop drinking alcohol because it makes them ill.

It is not a problem of getting drunk, as sensitivity to alcohol in AOPVFS can be marked. One glass of wine, a couple of beers or a whisky will, even in formerly quite heavy drinkers, produce symptoms of a profound hangover, which can last for several days. Most of the symptoms are confined to the central nervous system, and to the head in particular, but gastro-intestinal problems, if present, can worsen. There is not often a deterioration of the muscle symptoms.

We know of many situations and factors that worsen AOPVFS, such as intercurrent infection and excessive physical activity, but here we have a simple chemical substance which makes people ill, and within that statement possibly lies a great deal of understanding of some of the biochemistry involved in AOPVFS.

For example, it is clear that if one could identify the offending chemical or chemicals that are involved in the process of making the symptoms worse there must be a substance available that could block that effect, and so one could devise a drug that could improve the symptoms. It is thus important to find the chemical in alcoholic beverages that upsets people.

At the time of writing this book I have already begun some tests, based on trying to identify precisely what types of drink people are avoiding. Some of the initial answers have made me think that it is not in fact alcohol that is the culprit – there are a great number of chemical compounds in alcoholic beverages other than ethyl alcohol (C_2H_5OH).

Highest on the list are French red wines, then beer, lagers and last of all the spirits, with the possible exception of brandy, which seemed not to be causing many problems. This list suggested to me that it is not just the alcoholic content that might be incriminated, so I started to look into this a little further.

With the kind help of the husband of one of my patients, who acquired for me one litre of biochemically pure ethyl alcohol, I started to give people who expressed an alcohol sensitivity a 'wee dram' amounting to some 15ccs. I asked the patients to mix this with three times the volume of orange juice or blackcurrant, or some suitable alternative, and this would then give them a drink equivalent to a double scotch or a large glass of wine. I then asked them to drop me a note to tell me how they got on, and so far nobody has expressed any deleterious effects. So it initially appears that there is something else involved, and it seems to me that the most likely substances are the pressor and neuro-transmittor amines.

There are very few remedies or medications that improve the symptomatology of AOPVFS, but for a great number of years medicine has claimed that this disease is psychiatrically rather than organically based. Psychiatrists thus prescribe anti-depressants quite frequently, as they perceive this disease to be an aberrant depressive illness, and claim that patients get better with this form of treatment. In my experience, patients do indeed tend to improve, firstly because they suffer from a naturally fluctuating process that will get better anyway, and secondly because the majority of anti-depressants of all types are based upon the alteration of concentration of the monoamines in the central nervous system.

The central nervous system consists of the brain and the spinal cord and within this structure are many brain cells called neurones, which 'talk' to each other using chemicals. Neurones are electrically excitable cells that one could liken to an octopus; the body of the octopus would represent the body of the cell (neurone) and the arms of the octopus the axons of the nerve cell.

These axons are in some cases quite long and they form the basis of communication, spreading out to reach the arm or body of a neighbouring nerve cell. However, they do not quite touch – there is always a little gap, known as a synapse. In order to communicate a nerve cell sends a small electrical current down its arm and when this arrives at the synapse it causes the release of a chemical which passes across the synapse and stimulates the production of an electrical current on the other side. This electrical current then passes down a neighbouring cell's arm, or its body, and along another arm to another nerve cell, and so on.

There are many different sorts of synapses and many different chemicals involved, but the majority of the latter are monoamines, for example adrenaline, noradrenaline, and GABA etc. All of these substances are collectively know as neuro-transmittors and it has been demonstrated that there are significant alterations in their concentration in people who are depressed, anxious, obsessional or phobic. Antidepressants are therefore designed to alter the level of these chemicals within the central nervous system.

I believe that in AOPVFS there is a link between sensitivity to alcoholic beverages and the improvement noted with antidepressants, and this would be because both alcoholic drinks and antidepressants alter the concentration of monoamines in the central nervous system. The monoamines found in alcoholic drinks are the same as, or certainly resemble, those found as neuro-transmittors, and this explains why swallowing a greater or lesser amount of neuro-transmittor in your drink might make you feel ill.

I intend to expand on this by finding out precisely what chemicals are present in a decent bottle of Château Neuf du Pape, and then getting a suitable preparation made up and giving it to my patients to see what happens.

This is clearly important, because if I can identify the chemicals or substances that make people worse we may be able to develop a treatment programme that might get them better, either by avoidance of that substance, or by giving another medication that could block its effect. While I feel that this type of approach would not be in any way curative, it would certainly help to alleviate the symptoms. There is a lot we can learn from the simple fact that the majority of AOPVFS patients can no longer enjoy their drink!

The M.E. Action Campaign

In 1986 some members of the M.E. Association became rather disillusioned with what they saw as being the sluggish approach of the Association as far as publicity was concerned. They formed another group (later to become a registered charity) called the M.E. Action Campaign, headed by several notable people including Clare Francis as President, Jimmy Hood MP,

Melvyn Bragg, Leslie Kenton and Martin Lev. Their aim was to produce an action campaign to bring the plight of the M.E. sufferer to the attention of the general population and also of Parliament and I believe they did this very effectively, with benefit to all M.E. patients.

Having said that, I am extremely sceptical of the validity of the hypothesis they have developed about M.E. and I feel that it may bring the M.E. sufferer and the M.E. Association into disrepute and into conflict with the medical profession as a whole.

This hypothesis is that M.E. is caused by a toxic colon. Their point of view is that they have considered this theory very carefully and, although it is a controversial one for which they have no scientific proof, they feel that the evidence available is sufficiently convincing for them to publicize their ideas.

Their belief is that the presence of persistent enterovirus infection, candida and possible persistent bacterial infection in the gut, coupled with irritable bowel syndrome, points to something very wrong in the colon, leading to the fermentation of toxic products and the build-up of mucus and old faecal matter glued to the colon wall. On this basis, they point out some hopes for improvement or cure by 'cleaning old toxic matter out of the colon by colonic irrigation'.

I have pointed out my dismay at these ideas to the M.E. Action Campaign to no avail. My view is that this line of treatment is not just ill-advised but is positively dangerous.

Alternative treatments

There are many alternative treatments easily available today and, while some are of dubious value and exorbitant cost, others may offer some degree of relief to the patient – even if only on the grounds that taking an active approach to one's illness can have a therapeutic effect.

The Alexander Technique is a long-established and reputable treatment which is found on the curricula of many drama and music colleges. It is based on the theory that a two-year-old child has perfect balance which is subsequently lost through misuse of the body; muscles become tense through unnecessary abuse, setting up chain reactions throughout the system. For example, an actor may, through nervous tension, hunch his shoulders slightly when going on stage; this uses unnecessary energy and causes the neck and shoulders to become stiff and sore. Because of its emphasis on reducing wasted energy expenditure and stress on the muscular system, the Alexander Technique may well be helpful to M.E. sufferers.

Non-demanding and pleasant alternative remedies include aromatherapy and reflexology. Slightly more energetic, but again designed to alleviate stress, is yoga.

However, the most well-regarded of alternative treatments available is acupuncture. This has been reported as helping some people with ΛOPVFS and M.E. and it is worth considering it as a means of alleviating the symptomatology – I do not think anybody who practices acupuncture would claim that it can reduce the length of the disease process. Its primary role would be for the relief of pain such as headache and muscle ache; whether or not it can, as some of its advocates claim, improve the immune system is less certain.

Acupuncture is an ancient medicine and my view is that anything that lasts for two thousand years simply has to be effective. My own medicine is very untried in comparison, and whereas the knowledge I learnt when I left University is now obsolete, acupuncture has remained unaltered for centuries.

Acupuncture is the art of placing very fine needles into various points of the body; they are either left untouched, twiddled by hand, or vibrated with an electrical current. Sometimes smouldering herbs are applied to the needle to conduct heat down into the tissues; this is known as moxibustion.

The needles are placed along lines called meridians that are drawn over the anatomy and it is believed that these form lines of communication to various parts of the body. Stimulating the meridian lines can alter the body's response to pain and disease. Nobody knows how acupuncture works, but it is thought that various neuro-transmittors within the central nervous system are affected and chemicals called endorphines are released. Endorphines are morphine-like substances which can alter, usually by reduction, the perception of pain.

You should only consult a fully qualified acupuncturist who will have trained for many years; some practitioners have only done an abbreviated course and these should be avoided. Write to the Acupuncture Association and Register (see p. 242) for the name of a practitioner in your area.

Acupuncture is not a painful procedure and, while many people are alarmed at the prospect of having needles stuck into them, the needles are very fine and are only inserted a little way. Some acupuncturists use fresh needles for every patient, while others sterilize and reuse them. If you are worried about the possible transmission of disease, discuss with the practitioner what sterilization techniques he or she employs. You should expect to make three or four visits before you will know if the treatment is effective.

The candida problem

While many people believe that candida albicans has a role in the pathogenesis of AOPVFS and M.E. I am of a different opinion.

There are many different fatigue syndromes, and undoubtedly many causes for them. Candida may well cause a fatigue syndrome, but I cannot see its relationship with slow onset M.E. or AOPVFS, which are very specific disorders.

My disease definition of AOPVFS is that patients were formerly well and currently have no other particular diseases, and there is no indication that there are any predisposing factors to the development of candida. Those who are protagonists of the candida theory say that there is an increased intake of antibiotics in patients with AOPVFS and this is undoubtedly so in the initial phase of those complaining of upper respiratory tract infection. However, I do not think it has anything to do with the initiation of the disease, as 50 per cent of those with AOPVFS have never been given an antibiotic for their initial infection.

The oral contraceptive pill is suggested as another predisposing factor to candidiasis, yet only 5 per cent of my patients were taking it at the same time they contracted the disease or within one year preceding it. None of my patients was taking immuno-suppressive drugs such as steroids.

Supporters of the candida hypothesis continually refer to profound 'immune dysfunction' as being responsible for candida as well, but I do not have any evidence that the immune system is grossly disturbed, as one might find in AIDS. Consequently, I do not see any indication to evoke candida as a causative agent.

What is candida albicans?

Candida albicans is a yeast, and in its normal non-invasive form is a spherical spore, like a miniature football. We all have quite large quantities of this yeast all over the surface of our skin and especially in the moist areas of the body including the mouth, anus and vagina. It also lies within the gastro-intestinal tract. In its resting spore-like state it is harmless, but in its active state starts to divide, multiply and produce finger-like protrusions which branch. These branches travel rather like roots through the surface of the tissues, especially the mucous membranes; they then develop 'fruiting' bodies where more spores are reproduced to break off and spread elsewhere.

This growth and reproduction is constant, and occurs only in a very small way because the reproduction process is kept under control by many factors which include the natural immune responses, antibody production, chemicals that kill the yeast in its active phase, and a phenomenon called competitive inhibition. Within the mouth and vagina there are natural bacteria called commensals which line the mucous membrane and produce a defensive screen. They are responsible for the consumption of local nutrients, the production of acid, and the inhibition of the growth of other more harmful yeasts, fungi and bacteria.

These commensal bacteria maintain the status quo which, in this particular example, means the inhibition of candida. If something upsets this fine balance, the root growth and spore production increase and the candida becomes so prolific that it produces an infective process of its own called thrush. Babies quite frequently get it in the mouth, or it can cause nappy rash, and women commonly get it in the vagina, where it produces a white, irritating discharge.

The classical induction of thrush is seen after the administration of the broader spectrum antibiotics, such as Ampicillin or Amoxycillin. These cure the patient's infection but they also kill off a lot of the commensal bacteria within the mouth, the gut and the vagina, allowing oral or vaginal thrush to take over.

Other conditions which will allow thrush to increase are the local hormonal imbalances produced by the oral contraceptive pill, or a general lowering of body immunity or local mucous membrane resistance; it is not uncommon for someone run-down to get a recurrence of their thrush infection and it is prevalent in people with serious debilitating disorders such as chronic liver failure, chronic renal failure, the leukaemias, chronic tuberculosis and tumours. Almost certainly it is brought about here by a generalized systemic reduction in immune surveillance.

Many people never get it despite being given antibiotics; thrush infections tend to go for the very young, the very old, and women. Women who develop vaginal thrush find that it can recur simply as a result of intercourse, frictional changes within the mucous membrane presumably allowing an invasion by the locally found candida.

Yeasts live predominantly on sugars and carbohydrates and if one produces a larger amount of these substances locally this will encourage the overgrowth of candida. In diabetes there is frequently an abnormally raised blood sugar and mucous membrane sugar on which the candida thrives and becomes invasive.

The treatment of thrush is usually quite simple. Oral thrush in infants can be readily controlled with Nystatin oral drops and other anti-fungal preparations. In the adult more attention should be given to oral hygiene. Vaginal thrush is treated with anti-fungal topical medications, of which there are many, and by increasing the local acidity by lactobacilli applications or by substances that are acid in their own right. That is usually all that is required in the vast majority of thrush infection.

There are, however, a few medical diseases where thrush becomes invasive, passing through the mucous membrane and into the system as a whole. This indicates a very severe breakdown of immuno regulation and natural defence mechanisms, and such systemic candidiasis is quite frequently fatal in people who are in the final stages of AIDS or leukaemia, for example. Here massive doses of intravenous anti-fungal agents are required, and one could never eradicate systemic thrush by giving an anti-fungal agent by mouth.

Candida In AOPVFS and M.E.

While I do not believe that candida has any part to play in the initiation of AOPVFS and M.E., it may be that it contributes to some of the subsequent symptomatology. The case for this has been put to me by Dr Jonathan Brostoff, a consultant immunologist and allergist for whom I have a great deal of respect.

Dr Brostoff believes that candida could be responsible for some of the persistent symptoms such as gastro-intestinal disturbances and points out that a large number of people with M.E. and AOPVFS have an increase in vaginal discharge and candida, and pruritus ani ('itchy bum'). In his view it is possible that breakdown products from the candida within the gastro-intestinal system give rise to peripheral effects, such as headache and joint aches and pains. He feels that the anecdotal finding that patients improve on a low yeast, low sugar and low carbohydrate diet, coupled with Nystatin treatment, is important, and could indeed indicate that the symptomatology is aggravated by a candida infection. He does not believe, however, that any such regime will do anything to cure the underlying disease.

As a result of his advice I plan a study on the use of Nystatin in the management of M.E. symptomatology and I have already observed that patients on diets improve. However, Nystatin when given by mouth, either in tablet or powder form, is restricted to the gut and therefore only treats candida within the surface cells of the gastro-intestinal tract, and also within the lumen of the bowel itself. Those who suggest systemic candidiasis is implicated in M.E. are in error in saying they can treat this with Nystatin, which is not systemically absorbed.

The candida diet

Forbidden foods
Bread of any kind except 'Baking Powder Bread'. Yeasty buns, e.g. Chelsea, Bath, teacakes, rolls. Wimpies, hot-cross buns,

crumpets, hot dogs, doughnuts, pizzas, most oatcakes, cream crackers, twiglets

Bread sauce and stuffing containing breadcrumbs, breadcrumb coating on fish, fishcakes, fish fingers, rissoles, potato croquettes

Sausages, meat loaf, beefburgers, and other meat products containing bread

All cheese, ice cream, buttermilk, soured cream

Malted milk foods, e.g. Ovaltine, Horlicks

Synthetic creams, e.g. in pastries, eclairs etc.

All puddings, particularly bread pudding, queen of puddings, apple charlotte, bakewell tart

Wines, beers, lagers, cider, fruit juices

Grapes, sultanas, currants, plums, dates, prunes and anything containing these, e.g. fruit cake, mincemeat. All over-ripe fruit

Marmite, Bovril, Oxo, Bisto, soup powders, most tinned soups and stock cubes

Vinegar and all foods pickled in it or containing it, e.g. tomato ketchup, pickled onions, pickled beetroot, mayonnaise and salad cream, tartare sauce, soy sauce

Coleslaw, vegetable or potato salad

Raisin bran, muesli and sultana bran

All manufactured foods containing yeast extract or hydrolysed protein

All food with a high sugar content, e.g. sugar, jam, marmalade, sweets, chocolates, dried fruit

Because of probable sugar content these *may* have to be avoided: scones, any plain cakes, pastries, biscuits, fancy cakes or fruit tarts (not containing dried fruit)

Permitted foods

'Baking Powder Bread', soda bread, crispbreads, rice cakes

Ordinary sauces made with flour or cornflour

Cornflour crumbs, oatmeal coating and most batters

Any meat other than those forbidden plus fish or poultry

Eggs, milk, butter, cream, live yoghurt

Vegetable fats and oils, suet, dripping

Any fruit other than those forbidden – wash well before eating

Nuts

Fray Bentos stock cubes

Salt, pepper, herbs, spices, lemon juice

All vegetables, salads, potatoes

Cereals *not* containing dried fruit, sugar or malt – malt free cereals include Shredded Wheat, Cubs, Puffed Wheat and Rolled Oats

Coffee, tea, cocoa

It is recommended that while adhering to this diet one should also take some form of medication such as Nystatin to kill the candida already in the gastro-intestinal system.

There are several preparations of Nystatin, the most common being in tablet form. Alternatively, there is a powder marketed by Becpharm in 25 gram pots. This is not listed in Mimms but is, nevertheless, available on prescription.

There are therapists who believe that very large doses of Nystatin should initially be given, and that it is only at toxic levels that improvement occurs. This dosage should always be monitored medically by those who have experience of using it.

While I have my doubts as to the efficacy of an anti-candida diet and Nystatin therapy, they are neither dangerous nor expensive. Consequently, while I would not positively recommend this regime I would not condemn it either, unlike some of the more extreme suggestions of alternative therapy. The diet in itself, while nearly as boring as my exclusion diet, is certainly not medically a problem, and I understand that vitamin and mineral supplements can be taken without deleterious effects.

Your own doctor may be unwilling to prescribe Nystatin because it will cost the NHS money, and has not been proven to work. In this event you can obtain it by buying it privately.

If you do try the diet and Nystatin, I suggest you pursue it for three months. If you have noticed some improvement after that time, stop the diet and the Nystatin and see if you deteriorate. If you do, then obviously this is working for you and you should take them up again. You may in this case feel you would like more detailed advice on this type of therapy, in which case you should consult someone who has a good working knowledge of it or read one of the books devoted to the subject.

Useful addresses

M.E. Groups

United Kingdom
M.E. Association
PO Box 8
Stanford-le-Hope
Essex SS17 8EX
(Phone: 0375 642466)

M.E. Action Campaign
PO Box 1126
London
W3 ORY

Australia
G. Mulvany
Secretary
ANZMES Geraldton
93 Ainsworth Street
Geraldton
Western Australia 6350

Jenny Droop
Secretary
ANZMES Victoria
PO Box 7
Moonee Ponds
Victoria 3039

Val Southcombe
Secretary
ANZMES Perth
PO Box 293
West Perth
Western Australia 6005

Chrissy Finn
Secretary
ANZMES New South Wales
PO Box 645
Mona Vale
New South Wales 2103

Canada
Mrs K.M. Smith
PO Box 298
Kleinburg
Ontario
LOJ 1CO

Holland
Ms Marion Lescrauwaet
1106 DP Wamelplein 16
Amsterdam

New Zealand
ANZMAES
PO Box 35/429
Browns Bay
Auckland 10

ANZMES Inc.
PO Box 47–191
Ponsonby
Auckland 2

ANZMES Otago/Southland
PO Box 5412
Moray Place
Dunedin

Norway
Ellen Piro
Gullerasveien 14B
0386 Oslo 3

Papua New Guinea
Jean Hainsworth
New Guinea M.E. Support
PO Box 11
Ukarumpa
Via Lac

South Africa
Mrs Janine Shavell
66 Third Street
Lower-Houghton
Johannesburg

United States of America
American M.E. Society
PO Box 72
Skillman
New Jersey 08558

Chronic Fatigue Syndrome Society
PO Box 230108
Portland
Oregon 97223
(Phone: (503) 684 5261)

Treatment information

Acupuncture
The Acupuncture Association and Register
34 Alderney Street
London SW1V 4EU

Alexander Technique
Society of Teachers of Alexander Technique
10 London House
266 Fulham Road
London SW10

Aromatherapy
International Federation of Aromatherapists
46 Dalkeith Road
London SE21 8LS

Homoeopathy
British Homoeopathic Association
27a Devonshire Street
London W1N 1RJ

Reflexology
British Reflexology Association
Monks Orchard
Whitbourne
Worcester WR6 5RD

Yoga
British Wheel of Yoga
80 Leckhampton Road
Cheltenham
Glos. GL53 0BN

BIBLIOGRAPHY

A number of information leaflets are available from the M.E. Association (address above) including:

Smith, Dr D.G., *The Diagnostic Guidelines for Myalgic Encephalomyelitis*

Smith, Dr D.G., *The Management of M.E.*

Smith, Dr D.G., *Psychological and Psychiatric Problems arising from Post Viral Fatigue Syndrome*

Information leaflets about alternative theories and treatments are available from the M.E. Action Campaign (address above) including the hypothesis *Toxic Colon*.

Bibliography A

Further reading

Chaitow, Leon, *Candida Albicans*, Thorsons (1985)

Davies, Dr, & Stewart, Dr, *Nutritional Medicine*, Pan Books (1988)

Horn, Sandra, *Relaxation*, Thorsons (1986)

Ho-Yen, Darrel, *Better Recovery from Viral Illness*, Dodona Books, The Old School House, Kirkhill, Inverness IV5 7TE (second edition 1987)

Isaacson, Cheryl, *Yoga for all Ages*, Thorsons (1986)

Macintyre, Dr Anne, *M.E. Post Viral Fatigue Syndrome: How to Live With It*, Unwin Paperbacks (1989)

Mackarness, Dr R., *Not All in the Mind*, Pan Books (1985)

Maclarnon, K., *M.E. and Me*, Susan Abrahams Ltd (1988)

Marcus, Dr P., *Acupuncture: A Patient's Guide*, Thorsons (1984)

Melnick, Joseph, *Portraits of Viruses*, chapter on 'The Picornaviruses', Inter Virology 20 (1983) pp. 61–100

Ramsay, Dr A.M., *Post Viral Fatigue Syndrome – The Saga of Royal Free Disease*, Gower Medical (1986)

Shepherd, Dr C., *Living with M.E.*, William Heinemann (1989)

Vithoulkas, George, *Homeopathy: Medicine of the New Man*, Thorsons, (1985)

Wilkinson, Steve, *M.E. and You, A Survivor's Guide to Post-Viral Fatigue Syndrome*, Thorsons (1988)

Wookey, Celia, *Myalgic Encephalomyelitis: Post Viral Fatigue Syndrome and How To Cope With It*, Chapman and Hall (reprint 1988)

Zuckerman, A.J., *Principles and Practice of Clinical Virology*, John Wiley (1987)

Bibliography B
General medical articles and papers

Arnold *et al.*, 'Excessive Intracellular Acidosis of Skeletal Muscle on Exercise in a Patient with Post Viral Exhaustion/Fatigue Syndrome', *Lancet* (1984), Vol. 1, pp. 1367–9

Behan, Drs P & W.M. and Bell, Dr E., 'The Post Viral Fatigue Syndrome – An Analysis of Findings in 50 Cases', *Journal of Infection* (1985), Vol. 10, pp. 211–22

David, A.S., Wesselly, S. & Pelosi, A.J. 'Post Viral Fatigue Syndrome: Time for a New Approach', *British Medical Journal* (1989), Vol. 296 pp. 696ff

Gadian, *et al.*, Examination of Myopathy by PNMR', *Lancet* (1981), Vol. 11, pp. 774–5

Gray, J.A., 'Some Long-term Sequellae of Coxsackie B Virus Infection', *Journal of the Royal College of General Practitioners* (1983), Vol. 34, pp. 3–6

Keighley, B.D. & Bell, E.J., 'Sporadic Myalgic Encephalomyelitis in a Rural Practice', *Journal of the Royal College of General Practitioners* (1983) Vol. 33, pp. 339–41

Jamal, G.A. & Hansen, S. 'Electrophysiological Studies in the Post Viral Fatigue Syndrome', *Journal of Neurology, Neurosurgery and Psychiatry* (1985) Vol. 48, pp. 691–4

Schwartz *et al.*, 'Benign Post Infection Polymyositis', *British Medical Journal* (1978) Vol. 2, pp. 1256 7

Teahon *et el.*, Clinical Studies of the Post Viral Fatigue Syndrome with Special Reference to the Skeletal Muscle Function', *Clinical Science* (1988) Vol. 75, Suppl. 18, p. 45

Winbow, A., 'M.E. Presenting as a Psychiatric Illness', *British Journal of Clinical and Social Psychiatry*, (1986) Vol. 4, No. 2, pp. 1–3

Yousef, 'Post Viral Fatigue Syndrome'. *Update* (1 Jan 1989) pp. 33–7

Bibliography C
Specific enterovirus references

Archard *et al.*, 'Virus Aetiology of the Post Viral Fatigue Syndrome, Myalgic Encephalomyelitis: Persistence of Enterovirus RNA in Muscle', *Journal of Royal Society of Medicine* (June 1988) Vol. 81, pp. 326–9

Bowles *et al.*, 'Detection of Coxsackie B Virus – Specific Sequences in Myocardial Biopsies from Cases of Myocarditis and Dilated Cardiomyopathy', *Lancet* (1986) Vol. 1, pp. 1120–2

Dowsett, 'Human Enteroviral Infections', *Journal of Hospital Infection* (1988) Vol. 11, pp. 103–15

Gyorkey *et al.*, 'Coxsackie Virus Aggregates in Muscle Cells of a Polymyositis Patient', *Inter Virology* (1978) Vol. 10, pp. 69–77

Jehn *et al.*, 'Myositis and Myoglobinuria Associated with Enterovirus Echo 9 Infection', *Archives of Neurology* (1980) Vol. 37, pp. 457–8

Kadiry *et al.*, 'Analysis of Antigens in Circulating Immune Complexes of Patients with Coxsackie Infections'. *Supplement Progress in Brain Research* (1983) Vol. 59, pp. 61–7

Matteuci *et al.*, 'Group B Coxsackie Virus Readily Established Persistent Infections in Human Lymphoid Cell Lines', *Medical Journal of Virology* (1985) Vol. 56, pp. 651–4

McCartney *et al.*, 'Routine Use of u-Antibody Capture Elisa for the Seriological Diagnosis of Coxsackie B Virus Infections', *Journal of Medical Virology* (1986) Vol. 19, pp. 205–12

Tang *et al.*, 'Chronic Myopathy Associated with Coxsackie Virus

Type A9', *New England Journal of Medicine* (1975) Vol. 292, pp. 608–11

Bibliography D
Epstein Barr virus references

Editorial, 'EB or not EB? – That is the Question', *Journal of the American Medical Association* (1987) Vol. 257, No. 17, pp. 2335–6

Buchwald *et al.*, 'Frequency of Chronic Active Epstein Barr Virus Infection in a General Medical Practice', *Journal of the American Medical Association* (1 May 1987) Vol. 257, No. 17, pp. 2303–7

'Chronic EBV Disease: A Workshop', *Annals of International Medicine* (1985) Vol. 105, pp. 951–2

Borysiewicz, 'EBV Specific Immune Defects in Patients with Persistent Symptoms following Infectious Mononucleosis', *Quarterly Journal of Medicine – New Series* (1986) Vol. 58, No. 226, pp. 111–21

Caligiuri *et al.*, 'Phenotypic and Functional Deficiency of Natural Killer Cells in Patients with Chronic Fatigue Syndrome', *American Journal of Immunology* (1987) Vol. 139, No. 10, pp. 3306–13

Homes *et al.*, 'A Cluster of Patients with Chronic Mononucleosis-like Syndrome', *Journal of the American Medical Association* (1 May 1987) Vol. 257, No. 17, pp. 2297–2302

Hotchin *et al.*, 'Active EBV Infection in Post Viral Fatigue Syndrome', *Journal of Infection* (1989)

Rickinson, 'Chronic Symptomatic EBV Infections', *Immunology Today* (1987) Vol. 7, No. 1, pp. 13–14

Rickinson, 'The EBV as a Model of Virus-Host Interaction', *British Medical Bulletin* (1985) Vol. 41, No. 1, pp. 75–9

Strauss, 'The Chronic Mononucleosis Syndrome', *Journal of Infectious Diseases* (1988) Vol. 157, No. 3, pp. 405–12

Tobi *et al.*, 'Prolonged Atypical Illness Associated with Serological Evidence of Persistent EBV Infection', *Lancet* (1982) Vol. 1, pp. 61–4

Bibliography E

Reference 1. Behan et al. 'The Post Viral Fatigue Syndrome'. Analysis of the findings in 50 cases. *The Royal Society for the Study of Infection* 1985 (10, 211–222)

Reference 2. Jamal and Hanson Electro 'Physiological Studies in the Post Viral Fatigue Syndrome.' *Journal of Neurology, Neuro Surgery and Psychiatry 1985*: 48: 691–694

Reference 3. Arnold Radda Bore et al. *The Lancet.* Saturday 23 June 1984 1,367–1, 369

Reference 4. Waggonmakers Cokley and Edward 'The Metabolic Consequences of Reproduced Habitual Activities in Patients with Muscle Pain and Disease'. *Ergonomics* 1988: 31: 1, 519–1,527

Reference 5. Waggonmakers A.J. Cokley J.H. Edwards R.H. 'The Metabolic Consequences of Reduced Habitual Activities in Patients with Muscle Pain and Disease'. *Ergonomics* 1988; 31: 1, 519–1, 527

Reference 6.
Lloyd, Hales and Gandevia. 'Muscle Strength, Endurance and Recovery in the Post Infection Fatigue Syndrome'. *Journal of Neurology, Neurosurgery, and Psychiatry*, 1988; 51; 1, 316–1, 322.

Reference 7. Archard, Behan, Bell et al 'Virus Etiology of the Post Viral Fatigue Syndrome Myalgic Encephalomyelitis: Persistence of Enterovirus RNA in Muscle and its Correlation with Elevated Creatine Kinase Values'. *Journal of the Royal Society of Medicine.* June 1988 Vol 81. p.326–29

Reference 8. Cunningham, Bowles, Lane et al 'Persistence of Enteroviral RNA in Chronic Fatigue Syndrome is Associated with the abnormal Production of Equal Amounts of Positive and Negative Strands of Enteroviral RNA'. *Journal of General Virology* (1990, 71, 1,399–1, 402)

Reference 9. Miller, Carmichael, Calder et al 'Antibody to Coxsackie B Virus in Diagnosis of Post Viral Fatigue Syndrome'. *BMJ* 1991; 302: 140–143.

Bibliography F

Reference 1: Cunningham, L. Bowles, N.E. Lane, R.J.M. et al. 'Persistence of Enteroviral RNA in Chronic Fatigue Syndrome is Associated with the abnormal production of equal amounts of positive and negative strands of enteroviral RNA.' *Journal of General Virology* 1990 71, 1,393–1, 402.

Reference 2: Holmes, G.P. et al 'Chronic Fatigue Syndrome: A working case definition'. *Annals of internal medicine* (U.S.A.) 1988; 108:387–389.

INDEX